THE MIND INSIDE YANG STYLE TAI CHI

Lao Liu Lu 22-Posture Short Form

THE MIND INSIDE YANG STYLE TAI CHI

Lao Liu Lu 22-Posture Short Form

Henry Zhuang

YMAA Publication Center
Wolfeboro, NH USA

YMAA Publication Center, Inc.
Main Office:
PO Box 480
Wolfeboro, New Hampshire 03894
1-800-669-8892 • info@ymaa.com • www.ymaa.com

ISBN: 9781594393532 (print) • ISBN: 9781594393549 (ebook)

Copyright © 2016 by Yinghao (Henry) Zhuang
Edited by Leslie Takao
Cover design by Axie Breen
Photos by the author unless noted otherwise

10 9 8 7 6 5 4 3 2 1

Publisher's Cataloging in Publication

Names:
Zhuang, Henry.

Title:
The mind inside Yang style tai chi : lao liu lu 22-posture short form / Henry Zhuang. --

Description:
Wolfeboro, NH USA : YMAA Publication Center, [2016] | Includes bibliographical references, glossary and index. | Contents: Introduction of Yang-style lao liu lu taijiquan -- The mind approach of Yang-style lao liu lu (twenty-two form) taijiquan.

Identifiers:
ISBN: 978-1-59439-353-2 (print) | 978-1-59439-354-9 (ebook)

Subjects:
LCSH: Tai chi. | Tai chi--Psychological aspects. | Tai chi--Health aspects. | Yang, Chenfu, 1883-1936. | Mind and body. | Body-mind centering. | Qi (Chinese philosophy) | Martial arts. | BISAC: SPORTS & RECREATION / Martial Arts & Self-Defense. | BODY, MIND & SPIRIT / Healing / Energy (Qigong, Reiki, Polarity) | HEALTH & FITNESS / Exercise.

Classification:

LCC: GV504 .Z584 2016 | DDC: 613.7/148--dc23

Printed in Canada

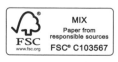

This book is dedicated to World Tai Chi Day.

修行太放鬆可以做為

修煉大手印之前行

雪漠

二三·十二·廿二

Learning and practicing taijiquan can serve as the preparation of learning Mahamudra.

Xue Mo

Dec. 12, 2012

Xue Mo is a famous Chinese writer, the vice chairman of Gansu Authors Guild, and a research expert of Mahamudra. He is known as the "father of contemporary Mahamudra research."

Editorial Notes

Romanization of Chinese Words

The interior of this book primarily uses the Pinyin romanization system of Chinese to English. In some instances, a more popular word may be used as an aid for reader convenience, such as "tai chi" in place of the Pinyin spelling, taiji. Pinyin is standard in the People's Republic of China and in several world organizations, including the United Nations. Pinyin, which was introduced in China in the 1950s, replaces the older Wade-Giles and Yale systems.

Some common conversions are found in the following:

Pinyin	Also spelled as	Pronunciation
qi	chi	chē
qigong	chi kung	chē gōng
qin na	chin na	chǐn nǎ
gongfu	kung fu	gōng foo
taijiquan	tai chi chuan	tī jē chǔén

For more information, please refer to *The People's Republic of China: Administrative Atlas*, *The Reform of the Chinese Written Language*, or a contemporary manual of style.

Formats and Treatment of Chinese Words

Transliterations are provided in the references: for example, *Five Animal Sport* (*Wu Qin Xi*, 五禽戲). Chinese persons' names are mostly presented in their more popular English spelling. Capitalization is according to the Chicago Manual of Style 16th edition. The author or publisher may use a specific spelling or capitalization in respect to the living or deceased person. For example, Cheng, Man-ch'ing can be written as Zheng Manqing.

Contents

Editorial Notes   xiii

Foreword   xvii

Chapter 1

Introduction of Yang-Style Lao Liu Lu Taijiquan   1

1-1.   Origin and Inheritance   1

1-2.   The Features of Yang-Style Lao Liu Lu   8

1-3.   Mind Approach in Practicing Taijiquan   8

1-4.   Key Factors of Mind Approach in Practicing Taijiquan   9

Chapter 2

The Mind Approach of Yang-Style Lao Liu Lu (Twenty-Two Form) Taijiquan   37

2-1.   Preparation Form   37

2-2.   List of Yang-Style Lao Liu Lu Forms   41

2-3.   Yang-Style Lao Liu Lu Complete Form   42

Glossary   207

Index   213

About Henry Zhuang   215

Foreword

This book was compiled by my friend Henry Zhuang. Taijiquan, a Chinese wushu, is the essence of five thousand years of Chinese culture. It is a reflection of the Chinese understanding that everything in the world consists of positive and negative materials. Taiji is integrity, the quality of being a gentleman, like Dao models itself after nature and the created universe carries the yin at its back and yang in front. Use the mind approach to practice, the mind to run the qi, and let qi move the body. With both the mind and body following the intent, one can prolong life and develop wisdom.

Huang Zhao Qiang
Chairman of Shanghai Wushu

Chapter 1

Introduction of Yang-Style Lao Liu Lu Taijiquan

1-1. Origin and Inheritance

In the time of Qing dynasty, taijiquan was quite popular in the royal palace due to Prince Pu Lun Bei Zi, a man of great power and wealth, who appreciated the fighting technique of Yang-style taijiquan. He recognized the martial applications disguised in the slow, graceful movements, as if there were needles hidden, wrapped in cotton. He invited Yang Jian Hou (third son of Yang Lu Chan—creating master of Yang-style taijiquan) into his mansion to teach and offered generous reward and favor, which influenced the Yang family to share their secrets of gongfu and taijiquan and to teach the traditional internal power that is usually called "Lao Liu Lu" or "Old Six Routines." However, it was Wang Chong Lu, a housekeeper and servant of Prince Lun, and his son who actually went into deep study and developed the deep understanding needed to inherit the internal power and technique. This became the bloodline thriving in the capital for the internal power and mind approach.

It is said, Wang Chong Lu, when formally acknowledging Yang as master, was instructed by Yang, "What I teach you [the mind approach of the internal power] shall not be released outside, except to your son. That is the Yangs' livelihood, and you do not want to ruin [it]." Wang and his son kept their word and never released any of the secrets of the mind approach of internal power. It was not until the 1990s, the third anniversary of Wang Yong Quan's passing, that *True Essence of Yang Style Taijiquan* was released to the public. In it he described, in detail, the essence of Yang-style Lao Liu Lu. It is a true classic of Yang style, which is the great achievement and contribution of Wang Yong Quan in his later years.

In 1982 Wei Shu Ren was formally accepted as a disciple of Wang Yong Quan. Wei was an adept student and gained favor from Wang, and took the instruction left by Wang to write books and accept disciples to promote Yang style. *True Essence of Yang Style Taijiquan* and *Yang Jian Hou's Private Teaching of Authentic Internal Power* were published in 1999 and 2000 respectively. They revealed the true essence of Yang-style Lao Liu Lu, for which we are fortunate, as the art was endangered due to the veil of secrecy kept by the masters of previous generations. It is a great contribution for human health.

Key Representatives

Yang Jian—The Second-Generation Master, Creating Master of Lao Liu Lu

Yang Jian (1839–1918), style name Jian Hou and also known as Jinghu, was called Gentleman Three by people, and Old Gentleman in his later years. A style name was given to imply a particular virtue. Yang Jian Hou was born with a subtle tranquility, a nature recognized by his father, Yang Lu. This subtle tranquility is an ability to abide or rest in the natural mind, or in Buddhism, in the Buddha nature. Persons born with this subtle tranquility are prime material for Dao cultivation and practicing internal boxing. He believed it would be Yang Jian Hou who would take the lead in the Yang family.

When he was practicing gongfu with his father, he completed all of his father's teachings, including more than ten complete forms, swords and spears, internal and external power training, concealed weapons, and shooting. The painstaking training was unbearable for most people, but was the key to Yang's ultimate exquisite gongfu. His boxing style couples both strength and gentleness, which is truly the ultimate realm, with mastery of sword, saber, spear, and pole. Many martial artists from other schools, skilled at sword and saber, challenged Yang, and all were beaten as if they were flies brushed away with a fly whisk. He was also skilled at spear and pole, capable of applying all kinds of forces to the tip of the pole. Therefore, when other spear or pole martial artists confronted him, they were all thrown away. He was an expert in shooting as well, and accurate every time. With three or four stones at hand, he could shoot down birds of the same number. What was unbelievable was his skill of holding a bird in the open palm of his hand and through sensitivity to the bird's motion prevented it from flying away.

The internal power is difficult to acquire. It must be practiced with both qi and spirit. Taijiquan inherently can function as dao yin, a practice to develop qi. At a novice level, after a person is able to relax and open the hips and shoulders, he is able to exert a holistic force. Only Yang was different, he started to throw people with the light and agile force. The relaxed and sinking force is holistic. It is triggered from the foot, reaching the touch point instantly; the light and agile force is a holistic one with internal force, making the touch point feel gentle, while the empty force gives almost no feeling at the touch point.

Yang Jian Hou, on the basis of the "small form" of his father, Yang Lu Chan, considering the physical conditions of the learners and focusing on health first, revised the form into "middle form," with extended movement range and reserved battle technique, which meets the demand of health for old people. This is another advancing step for Yang-style taijiquan. Standing push-hands and si zheng shou (four cardinal directions) were created by Yang Jian Hou, who also set Yang-style da lu (big rollback) and moving si zheng shou.

Yang Jian Hou had three sons: first son, Yang Shaohou (also called Zhaoxiong or Meng Xiang); the second son, Yang Zhaoyuan, died an early death; the third son, Yang Chengfu (also called Yang Zhaoqing).

Wang Yongquan—Successor of Yang-Style Lao Liu Lu

Wang Yongquan (1904–1987), "Zai Shan" (on the mountain), was the former vice chairman of Beijing Wushu Association.

Wang's father, Wang Chonglu, was a disciple of Yang Jian Hou, who often taught Prince Pu Lun on Yang's behalf. Wang started learning with Yang Jian Hou and Yang Shaohou when he was seven. He was liked by the Yangs due to his strength, cleverness, and willingness to work hard to learn. In 1917 Yang Jian Hou appointed Yang Chengfu (his third son) to teach Wang Yongquan. Yang Chengfu wanted to take Wang to Shanghai in 1928. However, the Wang children were still too young for him to leave. Wang was there for more than ten years, watching, learning, and gaining an understanding of both physical and mental aspects of the art. He acquired the true essence of the internal power and strength, and attained a high level in push-hands. He stuck to the original way of practicing Lao Liu Lu in his last decades, which is different than what Yang Chengfu taught in Shanghai or other places.

In 1957, Wang Yongquan, representing Yang-style taijiquan, was selected to the Beijing Wushu Team to participate in the First

National Form Sports Contest, and was awarded second place in taijiquan ranking. He performed excellently in national contests afterward, which convinced many people to want to learn from him, but Wang turned down the requests because of his vow of not disclosing the Yang style to outsiders.

At the end of 1957, many well-known practitioners in the Beijing martial arts community gathered with the municipal sports committee for the Wushu Association Meeting. Among them were Cui Xiulin, Wang Xiachen, and Sun Jianyun. They asked Wang for the true essence of Yang style, but Wang refused to unveil the secret of Yang style publicly in the meeting. This demonstrated to the entire wushu world how he treasured the rare art of Yang style, and of his uprightness and honesty in refusing to disclose the secrets.

Fortunately, in the early eighties, when the true essence was disappearing, convinced by people he respected, Wang loosened the restrictions and started lecturing about taijiquan in the Chinese Academy of Social Sciences (CASS). He explained the theory with plans and steps, demonstrated push-hands, and publicized what he had learned to people who shared his interest.

In January 1986, the initial draft of *True Essence of Yang Style Taijiquan* was finished, told by Wang Yongquan and organized by his students Wei Shuren and Qi Yi. In 1990 the book was posthumously introduced to the public. Today it is a taijiquan classic describing the heart of Lao Liu Lu and helping people understand the true essence of Yang style. That was a great achievement and contribution by Wang.

In June 1987, People's Sport Publishing House made tapes of Wang's push hands technique. Although Wang could hardly stand, to the amazement of the audience, he was able to throw the opponent meters away, with profound internal power.

Wang's teaching principles are value internal power—the training of intent, qi, and spirit; virtue first—learning taiji not for fame or wealth, but for practicing the Dao. The features of the form are comfortable, pleasant, and unaffected. Practicing taiji should follow the Dao, which follows nature. He clearly pointed out that taijiquan includes two parts of gongfu: self-awareness and opponent awareness. Self-awareness is the gongfu of cultivating the inner qi, by relaxing, expanding, connecting, and emptying. Opponent awareness is the gongfu of fighting techniques that applies the taiji force upon the opponent, by sensing, testing, controlling, and releasing. He did not only inherit and go deep into the tradition, but also made creations and developments, making outstanding contributions to the cause of Chinese taijiquan.

The followers of Wang Yongquan include Zhu Huaiyuan, Sun Deshan, Zhang Guangling, Zhang Xiaoda, Gao Zhankui, Wang Pingfan, Zhao Shaoqin, Sun Gengfu, Ding Guanzhi, Sun Deming, Qi Yi, Liu Wanzhong, Wu Youwen, Zhang Wenjie, He Fengshan, Liu Jinyin, Wei Shuren, Lu Zhiming, etc.

In April 2006, the successors of Wang held a memorial for Master Wang Yongquan in Taihe Palace in the Forbidden City, after which Yongquan Taijiquan Research Council was founded in keeping with Wang's dying wish of saving and promoting his teaching of health preservation and fighting technique, and of spreading the Yang style to the world.

Wei Shuren—Third-Generation of Yang-Style Lao Liu Lu

Wei Shuren (1924–2012) was a famous Yang-style taijiquan master, and inheritor of taijiquan internal power secrets handed down from Yang Jian Hou.

Wei started to be extremely interested in taijiquan when he was young. For twenty-eight years, before meeting Wang, he learned two versions of taijiquan: twenty-four-form simplified and the eighty-eight-form that are promoted by the country. He also learned the first and second routines of Chen style, short saber of Yang-style taijiquan, taijiquan pair practice, taijiquan sword pair practice, and Wudang saber pair practice with Gai Dianxun, Jiang Yukun, and Liu Guitang.

When he was seventy, Wang Yongquan was invited to teach taijiquan at the Chinese Academy of Social Sciences (CASS). To dig deep in the true essence of Yang-style taijiquan, Qi Yi, head of Philosophy Institute of CASS, and Wang Pingfan, head of Literature Institute, discussed and decided to ask Wei Shuren to learn from Wang, and organize the theories and forms taught by Wang Yongquan. After Wei formally acknowledged Wang as his master, he learned and studied diligently to understand the internal force that comes from using the concept that "the intent leads and form follows" in Yang style and the subtleness of "connected opening and closing," and experienced the wonderful force applied in push-hands. His rapid improvement won Wang's favor. In 1990 Wei and Qi organized the book *True Essence of Yang Style Taijiquan* told by Wang Yongquan, and promoted the almost-lost art to society.

In 1992 Wei participated in the Taijiquan Push-Hands Exchange of Nine Provinces and Cities on behalf of Beijing Taijiquan Team, and won high praises from other participants with his pure Yang-style internal power and exquisite push-hands technique. In May of the same year, he was invited by Hunan Provincial Taijiquan Association to teach in Changsha, and honored as a senior consultant of the association. In 1994 he was invited to teach in Shou De Martial Arts in Australia, and honored as a Yang-style taijiquan master. In 1995 he went to teach in Melbourne, Australia. In 1996 he was invited by Taipei National Martial Arts to teach and for the premiere *of True Essence of Yang Style Taijiquan Sequel*. In 1998 he was invited by Wenzhou Wushu Association to teach in Wenzhou.

Wei Shuren, undertaking the dying wish of Wang Yongquan to share the art, has been writing books, teaching disciples, and promoting Lao Liu Lu. In 1999 the *True Essence of Yang Style Taijiquan* written by Wei was introduced to the public. In 2000, his *True Essence of Yang Style Taijiquan Internal Power Secret from Yang Jianhou* (disc and instructions) was also published. It systematically disclosed the subtleness of the mind approach of internal power and condensed the eighty-nine-form Lao Liu Lu into twenty-two forms, which had built the stairs to the taiji world for those studying the true essence of taijiquan.

1-2. The Features of Yang-Style Lao Liu Lu

Guide the qi with intent, which diffuses in the body, with upper and lower body following each other, opening and closing connected.

Wei Shuren's understanding of the true essence of taijiquan:

"The spirit is shown as a dot floating. Calm the mind and hold in the intent with the qi rising from the back. Hands and feet moving without knowing. This is where the subtleness lies."

1-3. Mind Approach in Practicing Taijiquan

This chapter is an assembly of the use of internal force and the theory of internal power from *The True Essence of Yang Style Taijiquan—Lecture Notes* by Wang Yongquan, *The True Essence of Yang Style Taijiquan* by Wei Shuren, and the experiences and inspirations of the author.

The mind approach we talk about is a way of practicing with one's heart (mind and intent) as the guidance. There are no fixed patterns or rules; however, the mind approach I present has its principle based on the following six points.

Six Points for the Mind Approach

Taijiquan consists of yin and yang, and shows yang as the form (body movements), with the existence of yin as the foundation (spirit, intent, and qi). The mind approach presents the mutual reinforcement of yin and yang, thus revealing the basic rule of taijiquan, with harmony both internally and externally.

The intent runs through the entire taijiquan practice. Every move is made by intent.

The process of the mind approach is to use intent to lead qi to trigger body form. Use the heart (mind and intent) to circulate qi; use qi to move the body, first in the heart, and then in the body.

Intent and qi are the rulers, leaders, and dominators; the body is ruled, led, and dominated. What is the standard when you talk about body and use? Intent and qi are the emperors, with bone and flesh as the ministers.

Emphasis on intent first can change the habit of using brute force, aid in getting rid of stiffness, and build flexibility. In other words, use intent instead of strength.

The "mind approach" is just a name; it is just a raft, which finishes its mission when it carries one to the opposite bank, with weak overcoming strong, and less strength winning over more strength.

1-4. Key Factors of Mind Approach in Practicing Taijiquan

Here are the key factors. (For more of this discussion, please see *The Mind Inside Tai Chi* [YMAA, 2015].)

Qi

Small ball and big mass of qi

Mid-perpendicular and the plumb

San guan (three gates)

Three circles of qi

Cross in the chest

Source of force

Look of the eyes

Taiji diagram and the yin and yang palms

Eight types of forces

Qi

The first element of mind approach in practicing taijiquan is qi. When related to heaven and earth, qi is the entity creating something out of nothing. When related to taijiquan, it is the agent for the intent to lead the form. This is the mechanism of qi, namely, the law of qi.

Intent—Qi—Form

All bodily movements in taijiquan are led and influenced by the intent and qi. The intent and qi change and function through the transitioning of bodily movements. In practicing, the body cannot be separated from the dominance of the intent and qi. It is mainly directed by the trend of the intent and qi, and controlled and coordinated by the spirit, intent, and qi.

For beginning taijiquan enthusiasts who want to enter the real world of taijiquan, a student must approach the practice of taijiquan as something more than an aerobic exercise. To learn the subtlety of the use of internal force and power, one must learn the mind approach of the internal power in which the inner qi is of major importance.

Small Qi Ball

Imagine there is a small qi ball in each hand, and try to feel its existence but without any influence of subjective ideas. It doesn't matter if there is no feeling at the beginning. Focus on the qi balls, which are round or nearly round, but do not focus on a specific shape, feel, color, or weight. You are not so much creating as you are observing and monitoring a small qi ball. The relationship with the small qi ball and the palm is that in every move, the palm sticks to the edge of the qi ball and follows the movement of the ball.

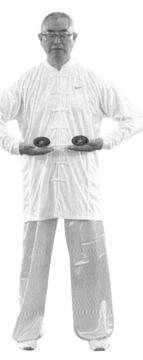

With the palms facing upward, imagine holding a small qi ball in each palm.

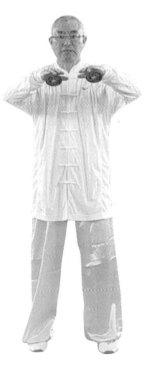

With the palms facing down-ward, imagine a small qi ball in each palm, as if the palms were adhering to the balls.

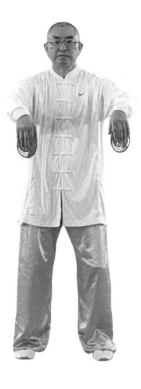

Imagine the small qi balls in the palms. The palms rise upward in front of the body before the arms stretch forward.

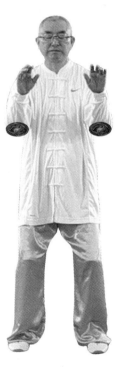

Imagine the small qi balls rolling from the palms, along the forearms, to the olecranons, the bony point of the elbow joint, before lowering the elbows.

Imagine the small qi balls at
the olecranons rolling back to the
palms along the forearms before
lowering the arms.

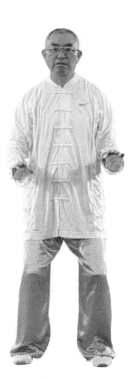

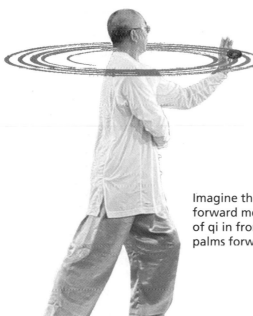

Imagine the small qi balls moving
forward merging into the circle
of qi in front before reaching the
palms forward.

Big Qi Ball Mass

After practicing and coming to understand the approach of using heart to control qi, and using qi to move body, I came up with the use of the mass. The big qi ball mass is an expansion and feeling of combining the small qi balls into one mass. Small qi balls can become big qi balls and big qi balls can break apart into small qi balls as the intent requires.

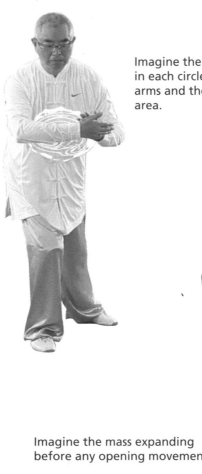

Imagine the qi diffusing around in each circle surrounded by the arms and thoracic-abdominal area.

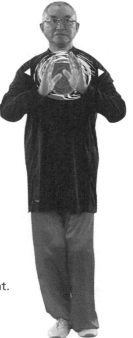

Imagine the mass expanding before any opening movement.

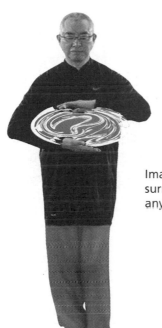

Imagine compressing the mass surrounding the body before any closing movement

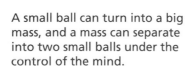

A small ball can turn into a big mass, and a mass can separate into two small balls under the control of the mind.

The Mid-Perpendicular

"The mid-perpendicular is an imaginary line traveling down through the center of the body. It cannot move up or down, only forward, backward, left, and right in fixed position. With its movement, the body can be in a straight line without leaning in any way and move the waist and hips horizontally with hand and foot in alignment in practicing. While the internal power is building up, the mid-perpendicular grows larger and the movements will be more agile" (*The True Essence of Yang Style Taijiquan*, by Wei Shuren).

The Plumb

Imagine there is a plumb in the body while practicing. "The plumb can swing in all directions, rotate, and raise and fall between the chest and the hips. In practicing, the brisk and agile turns and the swinging movements are all dependent on the plumb" (*The True Essence of Yang Style Taijiquan*, by Wei Shuren).

If you imagine a human as a bell, it shall be the outer form of a person. The plumb is a criterion for using the internal force. The corresponding swinging of the plumb causes the forward and backward movement. The turning of the body is caused by the turning of the plumb. Make sure the intent comes first followed by the form (or body), with the plumb swinging, connecting the legs, making the lower body light, agile, and steady.

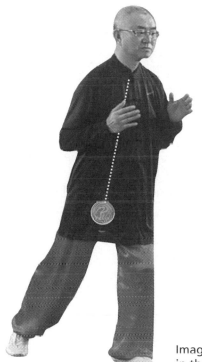

Imagine there is a plumb
in the body.

Rules

"Do not use the intent on both the mid-perpendicular and the plumb simultaneously. They do not appear to be used together. When using the intent on the mid-perpendicular, it appears instantly and disappears afterward. It is the same with the plumb" (*The True Essence of Yang Style Taijiquan*, by Wei Shuren).

San Guan (Three Gates)

The san guan (three gates) include weilu, jiaji, and yuzhen. Weilu is located at the lowest end of the spine, the midpoint between the apex of the coccyx and the anus. Jiaji is at the middle of the shoulder blades. Yuzhen is located on the back of the head that touches the pillow when you lie down. The san guan is a path of marrow for yang qi to travel up.

The Use of San Guan

The use of san guan includes vertical, leading up, leaning long, leaning forward long, and retreating. Using any of these is done with the inner qi traveling through the san guan in a straight line, led by the intent. The vertical and long san guan are the stretching out and drawing back of the spine. The long san guan is the opening created by suspending the head, relaxing weilu, and sinking to pull both ends to stretch the spine. The vertical san guan is the closing created by contracting the spine to resume the nature vertical status. The stretching out and drawing back of the spine is beneficial for the movements of the internal organs and preservation of health. It can also be used in fighting as a force from the back and the spine.

Vertical San Guan

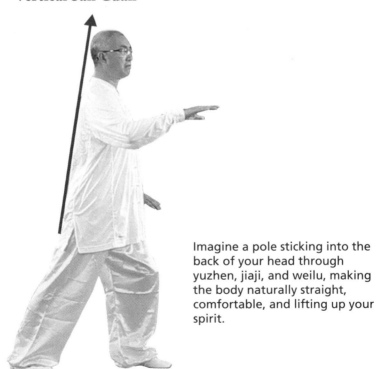

Imagine a pole sticking into the back of your head through yuzhen, jiaji, and weilu, making the body naturally straight, comfortable, and lifting up your spirit.

Leading Upward San Guan

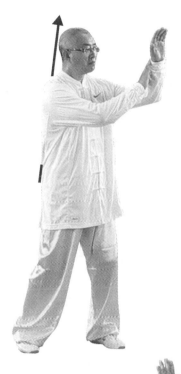

Imagine the san guan leading upward from the back of your head in a line, followed by the body stretching. After leading up, there will not be any heaviness or stiffness.

Leaning-Sideways San Guan

Imagine the san guan leaning sideways in a line, with a clear differentiation between the empty foot and the substantial foot. The arms stretch in opposite directions.

Leaning-Forward San Guan

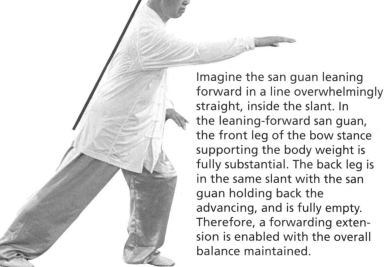

Imagine the san guan leaning forward in a line overwhelmingly straight, inside the slant. In the leaning-forward san guan, the front leg of the bow stance supporting the body weight is fully substantial. The back leg is in the same slant with the san guan holding back the advancing, and is fully empty. Therefore, a forwarding extension is enabled with the overall balance maintained.

Retreating San Guan

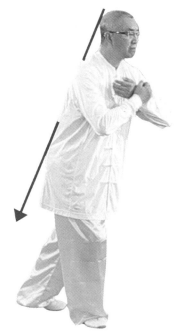

The intent of the san guan retreats through the weilu. Imagine a thin line penetrating through the san guan being pulled backward from the weilu, making the body move backward easily.

The Three Circles of Qi

The channel for expansion

Relax from up to down, head to toes. Then reverse the direction and relax from the waist and hips, the intent and qi expand around into shoulder, waist, and hip circles. When your gongfu is deeper, it will not only expand into the three flat circles, but also in all directions and then into a big mass of qi.

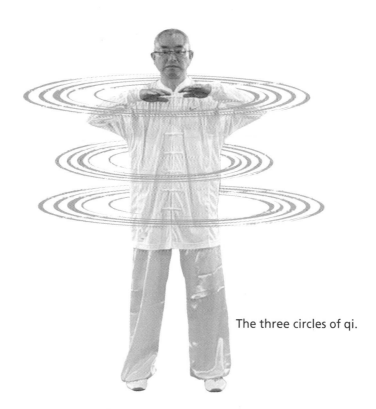

The three circles of qi.

Using intent to turn the waist circle comes first

The *Taijiquan Treatise* mentions controlling from the waist. While practicing, the left and right turns of the body are controlled by the waist. But trying to turn the waist directly would violate the principle of the intent first, and would make the body heavy and stiff. The waist should be empty. The left and right turns must be started with the intent turning the waist, which will then lead to the turn of the body, resulting in a light and agile body.

The Cross in Front of the Chest

While practicing, if you imagine a cross hanging in front of the chest, the shoulders would be even and straight, and the body would not tilt. Therefore, there are sayings like "pay attention to and study the purpose of every posture, and it will come to you naturally" and "the use is in the heart."

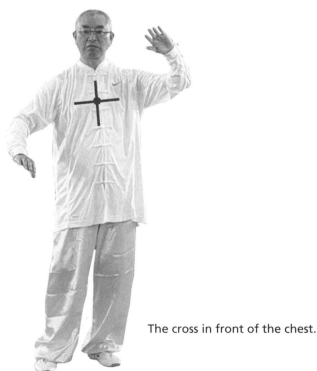

The cross in front of the chest.

The Source of Force

The source of force is where the internal force is generated. There are two sources, one at the middle between the shoulder blades. The other is on the upper palm at the root of the middle finger, when the internal power is at a higher level. That is what the ancient master meant by the source of force expands to the hands.

The use of the source of force

While practicing, the source of force on the back is the distribution center of the internal force all around the body. The internal force of every form shall be generated from it, which travels through the upper or lower lines of the arms to both hands.

The use of the source of force should be well under control. When it is needed in a form, the internal force will be triggered to reach the end, after which the source becomes empty at once. That is why the ancient masters talk about the subtleness of the source of force lies in it becoming instantly empty after delivery.

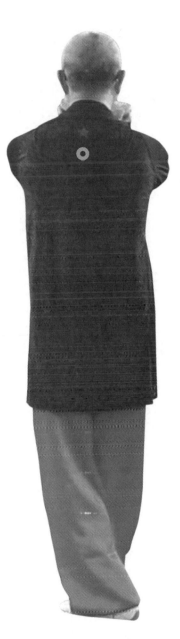

The source of force.

The conversion and changing between the forces also need to be done through the source of force. For example, to convert the four side forces into the four corner ones, one just needs to imagine a slight rotation of the cross on the source of force at the back without any body change, which is called "conversion between the sides and corners." When the power is improved and the source of force expands to the hands, the source on the hands is the same with that on the back.

Look of the Eyes

The look expresses the internal spirit and momentum, through the change of the range of the line of sight, matching the distribution of the intent, qi, and the postures. When one has grasped the upright bodywork with the neck relaxed, the head will be "empty," the eyes can naturally look without seeing, the ears can listen without hearing. The comfort of the head will make the internal spirit express on the face smoothly with a smile.

The use of the look

The use of the look needs to match the flow of the intent and qi, and the opening and closing, in and out of the movements, integrating the entire body to be in harmony with the spirit, intent, and qi, both internally and externally, up and down.

The controlling and releasing of the look have nothing to do with the opening and closing of them, but are related to tracks of the line of sight and the extending and retracting of qi led by the intent. When extending, the inner qi shoots out smoothly from the side corners of the eyes; when retracting, the qi of the eyes gathers to the middle from the vast field of vision and into the eyes from the midpoint of the eyes.

The leaving of the look must be accompanied with its entering, and vice versa. Thus, with the in and out in circulation can the use of the look of the eyes be enabled with yin inside yang, yang inside yin, yin and yang in harmony.

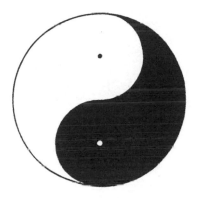

Yin and Yang Palms

To present the connotation of the taiji diagram, like the contradiction, mutual rooting, consuming, and transformation of yin and yang, and the rotary and round movement of the taiji boxers, we will use the yin and yang palms in the handwork. While practicing, one palm in the shape of the curved tile used on the roofs in China is at the upper front and the other is in the same shape following the base of the previous palm at the lower back. Imagine one of the palms holding a small black ball with a tiny white dot in the center, which is yang within yin; and the other palm, a small white ball with a tiny black dot in the center, which is yin within yang.

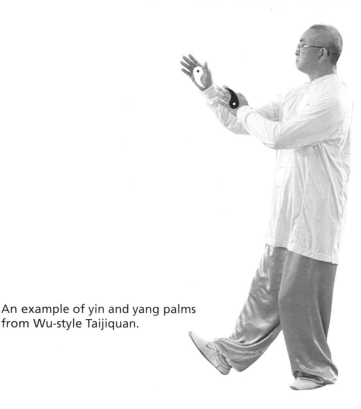

An example of yin and yang palms
from Wu-style Taijiquan.

Secret of the Eight Forces

(*Lecture Notes of Wu-Style Taijiquan,* by Wu Gongzao)

The eight forces are peng, liu, ji, an, cai, lie, zhou, and kao. Each
one of them has a special implication and use, which is interre-
lated and interdependent on the others to be functional.

In practicing, one needs to keep changing and combining the
eight forces in an organized way to provide a perfect internal force
needed for a posture without any deficiency. Meanwhile, only a
natural and controlled flow of movements in the form can enable
a smooth and easy use of the internal force (*The True Essence of
Yang Style Taijiquan,* by Yongquan Wang).

Peng

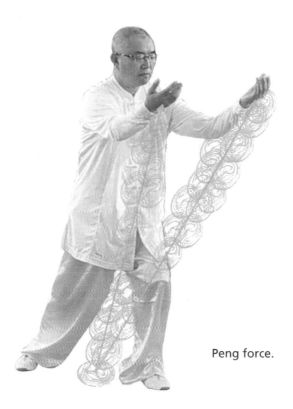

Peng force.

Peng (a floating upward force)

What is the meaning of peng? It is like floating a boat. First, allow the qi to fill the dan tian; second, suspend your head with a springlike force all over. Open and close in a suitable range. Even if it weighs a ton, making it float is no difficulty.

Liu (Lu)

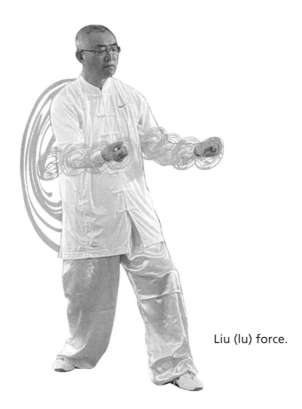

Liu (lu) force.

Liu (let it in and let it fall)

What is the meaning of liu? It is leading people to advance; follow this forward force, being agile without losing the head suspension. Emptiness comes naturally when its force is at its end; tossing or striking is at your will. Keep the center of your weight maintained so as not to be taken advantage of by others.

Ji

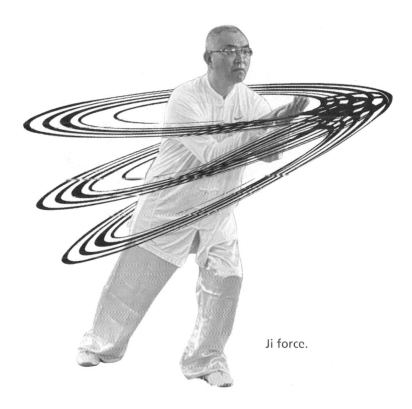

Ji force.

Ji (meeting up with accumulated momentum)

What is the meaning of ji? There are two ways of utilization; with a simple intent, meeting up and closing is in one movement. An indirect response is like a ball bouncing from a wall; also like a coin hitting a drum with a clang.

An

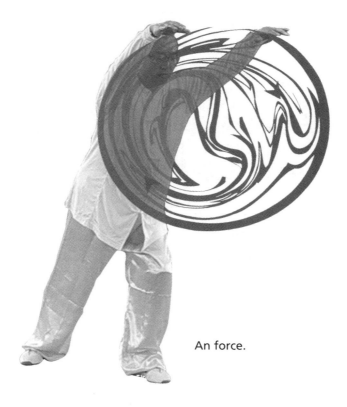

An force.

An (the ups and downs of the tide)

What is the meaning of an? It is like running water, unstoppable rapids, with firmness contained in softness. It splashes up when meeting something high and dashes down when meeting something low. Just like waves with ups and downs, it enters wherever there are openings.

Cai (Tsai)

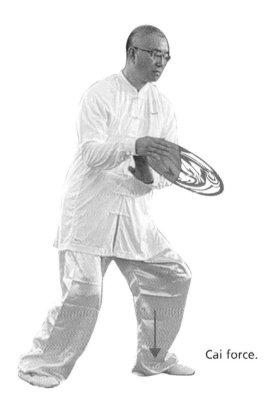

Cai force.

Cai (the force of pressing a lever)

What is the meaning of cai? It is like a counterweight on the beam. However strong or weak the strength is, it shall be clear only after weighing. If one asks theory, it lies in the leverage.

Lie

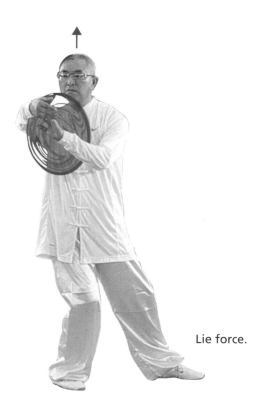

Lie force.

Lie (the force of slanted upward rotation)

What is the meaning of lie? It spins like a flying wheel. Anything on top is thrown far away. It is like an invisible whirl, twisting violently inside, which can sink a floating leaf in no time.

Zhou

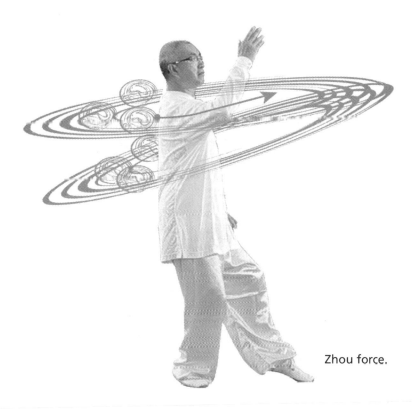

Zhou force.

Zhou (the force of lifting up)

What is the meaning of zhou? The use consists of five elements. Yin and yang separates up and down, clarifying substantial and insubstantial. It is unstoppable when connected, even more powerful when used as a hammer. The use of it is unlimited with mastery of the above six forces.

Kao

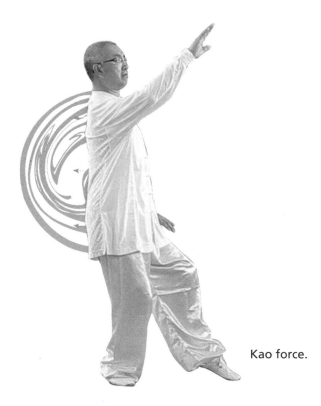

Kao force.

Kao (the force of leaning with your back and shoulders)

What is the meaning of kao? It has the back and shoulders. Use the shoulders in slant flying, with the help of the back. Once the advantage is gained, the opponent will crash like a smashed stone. But beware of the center of the weight, which if lost, everything would be in vain.

Stances

Bow Stance

Stand with one foot in front of the other. The front knee is bent. The knee should not extend beyond the front toe. Bend the back leg a little. The toes point diagonally to the front. The weight is more on the front leg.

Horse Stance

Take a step to the side, placing the feet parallel and about shoulder width or farther apart. Sit backward and bend the knees, with the thighs slightly above the horizontal level. Sink the hips and hold in the bottom. The upper body is straight. When there is more weight to the right, it is right horse stance, and when there is more weight to the left, it is left horse stance.

Squat Stance

Right squat stance. Bend the left leg with a downward force from the left knee and the weight on the left leg. Stretch the right leg sideways with the right foot holding the ground.

Left squat stance. Bend the right leg with a downward force on the right knee and the weight on the right leg. Stretch the left leg sideways with the left foot holding the ground.

Chapter 2

The Mind Approach of Yang-Style Lao Liu Lu (Twenty-Two Form) Taijiquan

2-1. Preparation Form

Wuji Stance—"Standing in the Sand"

Before you begin the sequence it is good to stand in wuji for a moment to focus your intent and your qi.

"Taiji is born from wuji." Wuji can be translated as "having no limits." Be calm and concentrated. Empty the mind. It starts to get obscured and merged. There is no yin or yang, you or others. Stand comfortably and steady as if you were a pole plugged into the sand. At the same time it feels like riding on a cloud in the sky. You and the earth as one.

- Head: Suspend the head. The *baihui* leads up to the sky, with the neck and head relaxed. The baihui is an important cavity located at the top of the head.

- Eyes: Control the look of the eyes. Converge the eyesight. Keep the eyes half closed.

- Tongue: The tongue touches the upper palate. Hold in the lower jaw.

- Chest: Open the chest and round the elbows. Relax the breasts (pectorals), feel the shoulders pulled back and down, and the elbows are sunk. The chest should be neutral and the back broadened and relaxed.

- Dantian: Trickle the qi into the *dantian*, which is located internally in the area below the belly button. That means to focus the intent in the dantian, with the lower abdomen relaxed and filled up. The *daimai* gradually spreads around. Do not apply any force or work against it. The daimai is the girdle/belt vessel, an energetic circle of qi around the hip area.

- Hips: Round the crotch, with the caudal vertebra pulled downward, with no upward or forward trend.

- Knees: Apply an upward intent on the knees. Relax the shank muscles.

- Ankles: Relax the ankles. No force should be attached to the ankles. Stand as if the feet are on the duckweed. Do not grab the ground with the toes, but focus the intent deep into the ground.

With a beginning in the mind, slightly open the eyes. Imagine, at a little more than three feet in front of the waist, a round dot gradually starting to shape out of nothing. Then it starts to ascend, with your visual focus until it reaches the eye level, from where it moves left and makes the left foot unintentionally yet naturally taking a step left to put a shoulder width between both feet.

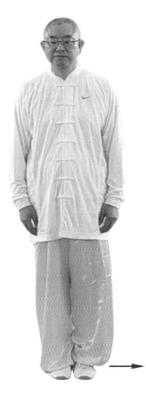

A beginning in the mind—
"Dao gives birth to one,
which is taiji."

Imagine the chest as two doors, with a small stone clipped in between. When they are opened backward by the intent, a sudden enlightenment appears. Meanwhile, the small stone falls into the lower abdomen, as if a stone tossed into the calm water, which starts rippling. When the inner qi diffuses into the back of the waist, it then keeps spreading sideways till the wrists start to *peng*. Peng is an action and a feeling of expansion. The qi keeps moving down to *huiyin*, a cavity located at the perineum. Then it moves from the upper third of the medial side of the thighs and along the *foot-tai yin spleen channel* on the medial side of the leg, through *sanyinjiao* on the medial side of the shanks. Then the qi flows along the *foot-shao yin kidney channel* through *taixi* and *rangu* on the medial side of your ankles down to *yongquan, on the bottom of the*

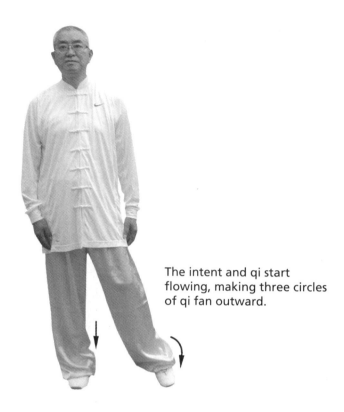

The intent and qi start flowing, making three circles of qi fan outward.

foot. Now it moves along the *gallbladder channel* from the lateral side of the ankles, through the lateral sides of the shanks, *and* the lateral sides of the knees, *continues* on the lateral sides of the thighs, then flows up the sides of the hips and *daimai.* The qi gathers at *mingmen* from both left and right and sinks into the *huiyin,* and then goes up to the midpoint between the hips (*dantian*). Then with the ascending line of the intent and qi as the center, use the intent to guide the inner qi to spread a circle of qi around the hips radiating about three feet. Meanwhile, the qi at the center of the hip circle keeps moving up to the waist and fans out into a waist circle radiating about three feet. The qi at the center of the waist circle keeps moving above the chest and spreads into a shoulder circle radiating about three feet.

2-2. List of Yang-Style Lao Liu Lu Forms

1. Commencing Form
2. Left and Right Parting the Wild Horse's Mane
3. White Crane Spreads Wings
4. Left and Right Brush Knee and Twist Step
5. Strum the Lute
6. Left and Right Retreat and Repulse the Monkey
7. Left and Right Grasp the Peacock's Tail
8. First, Second, and Third Open and Close Cloud Hands
9. Single Whip (Rolling, Rubbing, Folding, Grinding)
10. High Pat on Horse
11. Right Splitting Foot
12. Punch the Ears with Fists
13. Left Kick
14. Left and Right Fair Lady Works the Shuttle
15. Downward Posture
16. Rooster Stands on One Leg
17. Needle on Sea Floor
18. Fan Opens on the Back
19. Overturn and Throw Fist
20. Retreat, Deflect, Parry, and Punch
21. Seal and Close
22. The Cross Hands, Close into Taiji

2-3. Yang-Style Lao Liu Lu Complete Form

1. Commencing Form

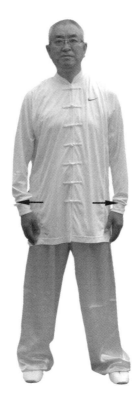

The inner qi goes down along the plumb to the middle of the crotch and spreads out forming the hip circle, with the wrists bulging. Imagine each palm holding a small qi ball which gently rises to the front of the chest led by the inner qi. (The direction you face when you begin the sequence is considered as south.)

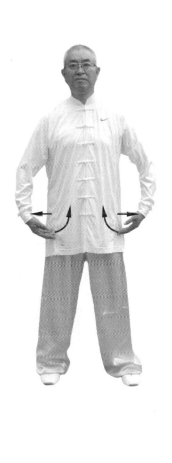

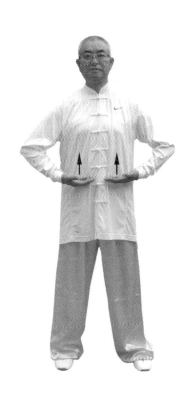

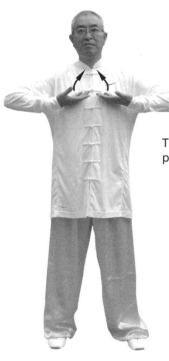

The two hands rotate inward, pressing the balls into the chest.

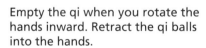

Empty the qi when you rotate the hands inward. Retract the qi balls into the hands.

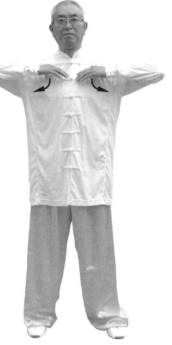

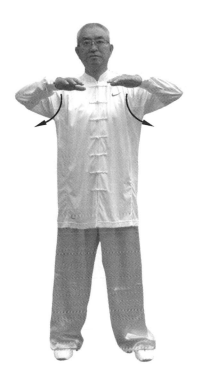

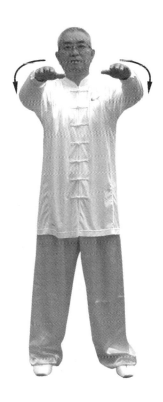

The palms adhere to the small balls facing downward, with inner qi diffusing into the arms from the source of force, which stretches forward.

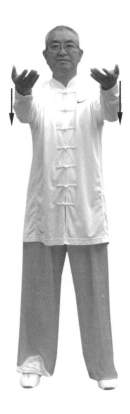

Resume the serenity of the mind. This feeling comes between practicing some patterns. You may need to instantly cut off the intent of the previous pattern. It is a moment between yin and yang. After a moment of quiet, a new intent starts to lead the new movement. Rotate the hands outward holding the qi balls.

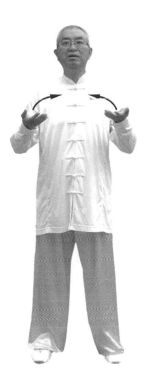

Slowly bend the elbows, closing in front of the chest to press the balls into the chest once more.

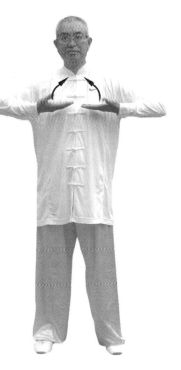

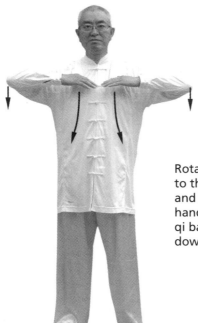

Rotate both hands inward close to the chest. Empty the hands and retract the balls into the hands. Then adhere to the small qi balls with the palms facing downward.

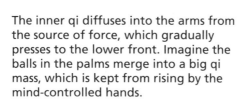

The inner qi diffuses into the arms from the source of force, which gradually presses to the lower front. Imagine the balls in the palms merge into a big qi mass, which is kept from rising by the mind-controlled hands.

2. Left and Right Parting the Wild Horse's Mane

Left Parting the Wild Horse's Mane

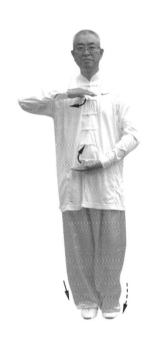

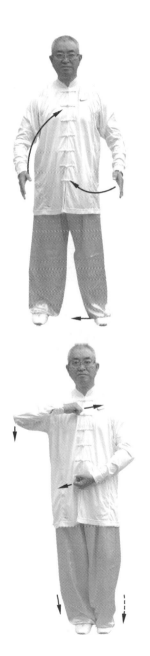

Imagine the qi mass in the palms rotates counterclockwise, with the left foot moving close to the right one, forming a substantial right leg and an insubstantial left leg. The right hand rises and the left one falls, triggered by the rotating mass, holding the qi mass in front of the chest and abdomen facing each other with one hand above and one below. Follow by grasping the small qi balls in the palm by gently closing into half-grasped fists facing each other.

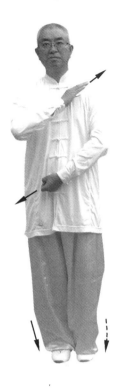

Send the small qi ball to the left
shoulder from the root of the
left middle finger, and from the root
of the left middle finger send the
other small qi ball to the lateral side
of the right hip. The qi mass diffuses
among the chest, abdomen, and
shoulders. The blending of the small
qi balls into a big qi ball makes the
entire body exert peng all around.

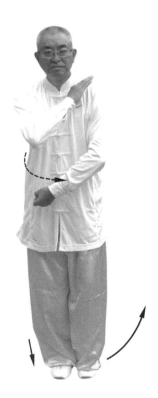

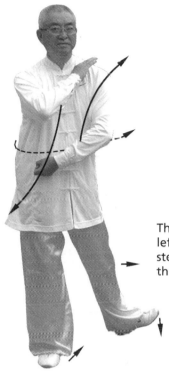

The waist circle turns left. Open the hips by stepping the left foot to the front left.

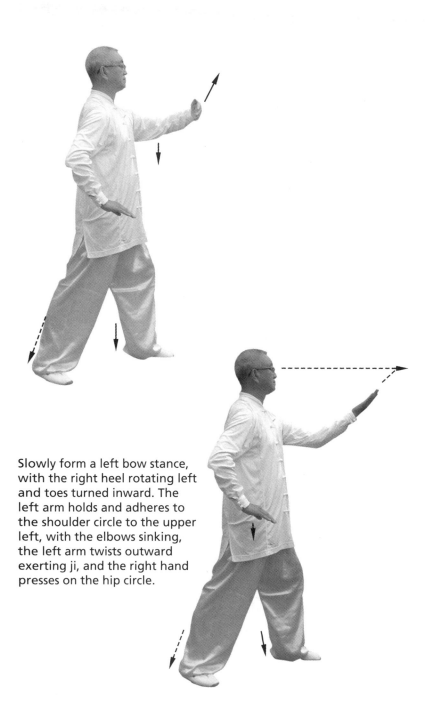

Slowly form a left bow stance, with the right heel rotating left and toes turned inward. The left arm holds and adheres to the shoulder circle to the upper left, with the elbows sinking, the left arm twists outward exerting ji, and the right hand presses on the hip circle.

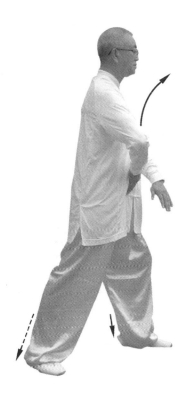

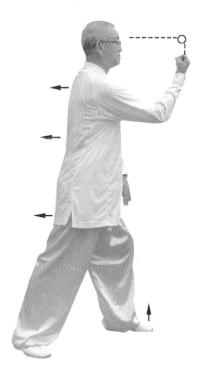

The right fist rotates with the torso, twisting and reaching forward through the chest. The root of the middle finger points forward and the left hand settles on the waist circle. This part of the movement is called approach the stars. "Approach the stars" is the upward movement of the fist. The fist moves as if it is going to approach the stars. When practicing, one should not only focus on the correct movement, which is fundamental, but also allow the intent to reach as far and deep as the imagination will take you.

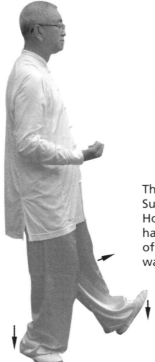

The plumb swings backward.
Substantialize the right foot.
Hold the small qi balls with
half-grasped fists and put the backs
of the fists against the sides of the
waist circle.

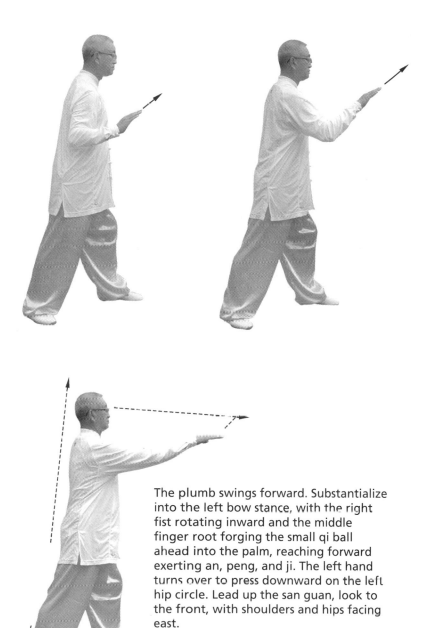

The plumb swings forward. Substantialize into the left bow stance, with the right fist rotating inward and the middle finger root forging the small qi ball ahead into the palm, reaching forward exerting an, peng, and ji. The left hand turns over to press downward on the left hip circle. Lead up the san guan, look to the front, with shoulders and hips facing east.

Right Parting the Horse's Mane

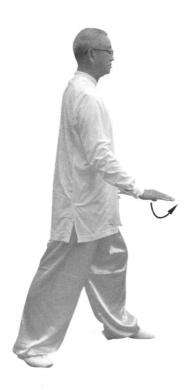

Sink the shoulders and elbows.
The right hand falls downward,
and the left hand lifts, holding
the waist circle with the palms.

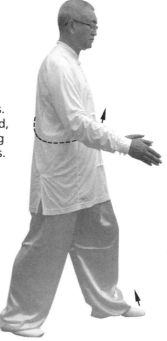

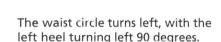

The waist circle turns left, with the
left heel turning left 90 degrees.

Imagine the mass in the palms rotate clockwise, with the right foot moving close to the
left one triggered by the rotating qi mass,
forming a substantial left leg and insubstantial right leg. The legs are slightly bent. The
right hand rises and the left one falls, triggered by the rotating mass. Hold the qi mass
in front of the chest and abdomen. The hands
face each other with one above and one
below. Follow by grasping the small qi balls
in the palm by gently closing the hands into
half-grasped fists. The fists face each other,
remaining in the same position. Shoulders and
hips face north.

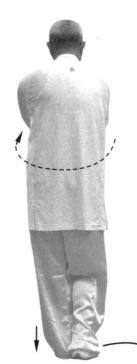

Send the small qi ball to the right shoulder from the root of the right middle finger, and send the other qi ball to the lateral side of the left hip from the root of the right middle finger. The mass diffuses among the chest, abdomen, and shoulders. The diffusion makes the entire body exert peng all around.

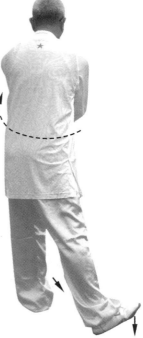

The waist circle turns right. Open the hips with the right foot stepping to the front right.

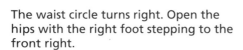

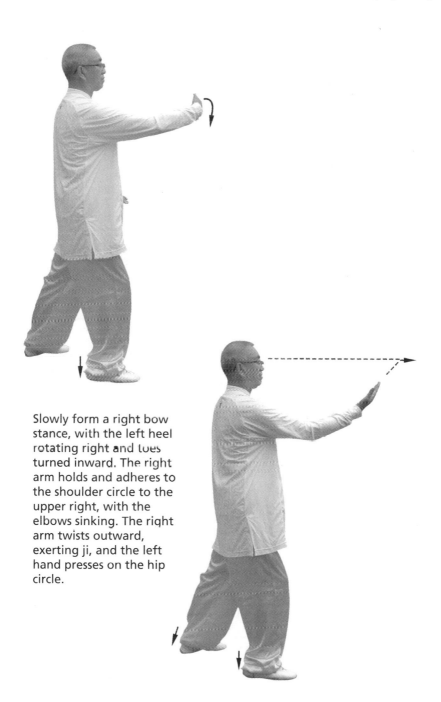

Slowly form a right bow stance, with the left heel rotating right and toes turned inward. The right arm holds and adheres to the shoulder circle to the upper right, with the elbows sinking. The right arm twists outward, exerting ji, and the left hand presses on the hip circle.

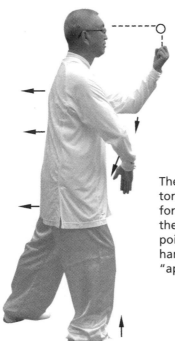

The left fist rotates with the torso, twisting and reaching forward through the chests, with the root of the middle finger pointing forward and the right hand settling on the waist circle, "approaching the stars."

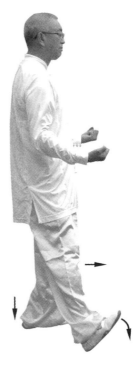

The plumb swings backward, with the left foot substantialized. Hold the small qi balls with half-grasped fists and put the back of the fist against the sides of the waist circle.

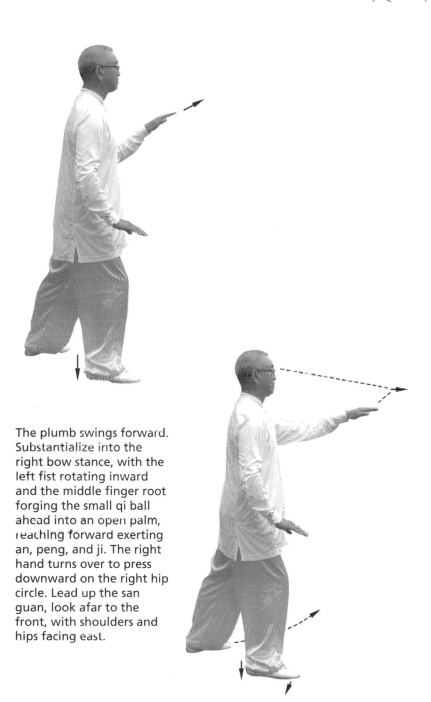

The plumb swings forward. Substantialize into the right bow stance, with the left fist rotating inward and the middle finger root forging the small qi ball ahead into an open palm, reaching forward exerting an, peng, and ji. The right hand turns over to press downward on the right hip circle. Lead up the san guan, look afar to the front, with shoulders and hips facing east.

3. White Crane Spreads Wings

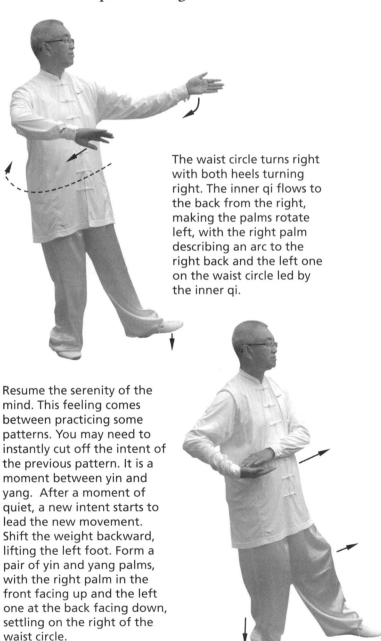

The waist circle turns right with both heels turning right. The inner qi flows to the back from the right, making the palms rotate left, with the right palm describing an arc to the right back and the left one on the waist circle led by the inner qi.

Resume the serenity of the mind. This feeling comes between practicing some patterns. You may need to instantly cut off the intent of the previous pattern. It is a moment between yin and yang. After a moment of quiet, a new intent starts to lead the new movement. Shift the weight backward, lifting the left foot. Form a pair of yin and yang palms, with the right palm in the front facing up and the left one at the back facing down, settling on the right of the waist circle.

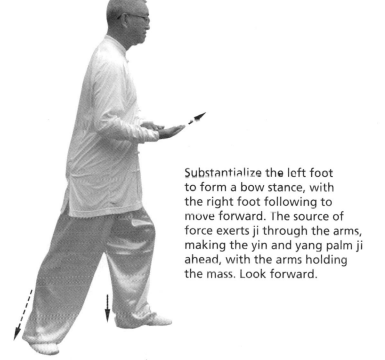

Substantialize the left foot to form a bow stance, with the right foot following to move forward. The source of force exerts ji through the arms, making the yin and yang palm ji ahead, with the arms holding the mass. Look forward.

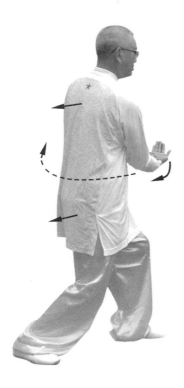

Move the weight back-
ward and substantialize the
right foot, with the waist
circle slightly turning right.
The source of force exerts lie,
making the yin and yang
palms lie to the right of the
shoulder circle, with the eyes
following.

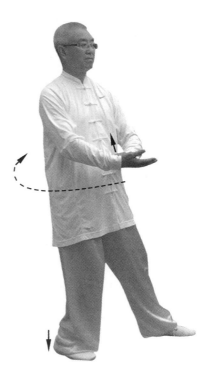

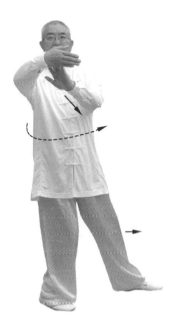

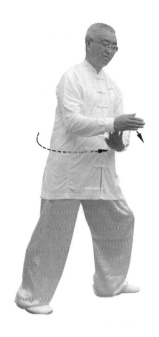

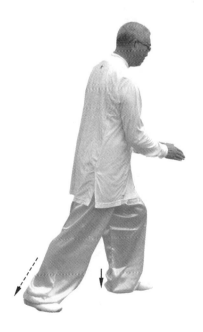

The source of force exerts cai, making the yin and yang palms move to the left hip circle with cai, to be in alignment with the left knee.

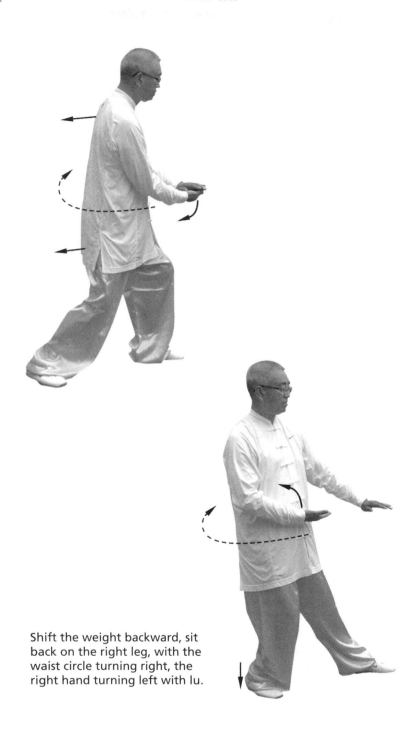

Shift the weight backward, sit back on the right leg, with the waist circle turning right, the right hand turning left with lu.

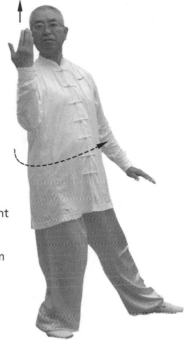

Keep exerting lu to the right of the waist circle and sink the elbow. Lead the right palm upward with the palm facing backward.

The waist circle turns left, while sitting back on the right leg. The left toes touch the ground insubstantially and the torso leans backward. The qi mass between the chest and back swells, separating the yin and yang palms. The left hand moves to the front left of the hip circle with cai exerted from the source of force, with the right hand rising up spirally exerting zhou through the right elbow, and kao through the left shoulder. Lead up the san guan and look forward.

4. Left and Right Brush Knee and Twist Step

Left Brush Knee and Twist Step

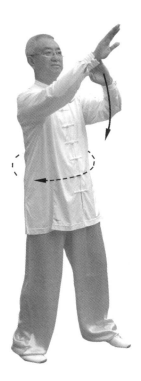

Substantialize the left foot, so the weight is centered. The left hand rises following the rising of the ball, with the tips of index finger, middle finger, and ring finger adhering and supporting at three cun lower than the back of the right wrist (i.e., contact by the palms).

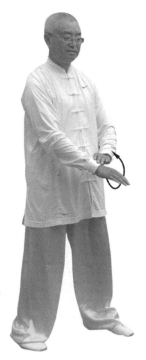

The left-hand fingers gently contact the right hand. They fall to the front of the crotch along the vertical line of the cross in front of the chest, following the falling of the balls of qi.

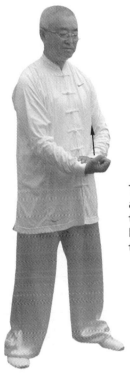

The right palm closes into a fist and turns inward with the back of the fist facing outward, and the left hand turning to be close to the inside of the right wrist.

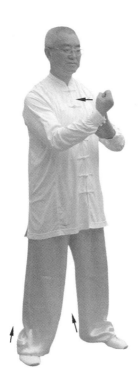

The right fist and left palm peng upward following the bouncing back of the inner qi from the floor. Bend the elbow, move forward with the balls of feet leaving the ground, the right fist at the cross center in front of the chest, drawing toward each other as if closing.

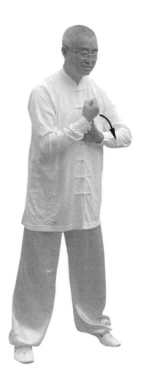

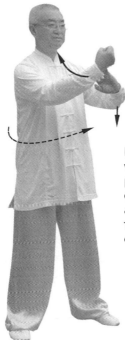

Resume the serenity of the mind, with the inner qi fanning outward, pushing the right fist to the shoulder circle. When straightening the elbow and retreating, the inner qi makes the torso and the hands repel as if opening.

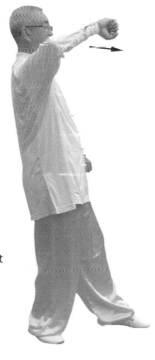

The waist circle turns left briskly, then right. Relax the shoulders and sink the elbows with the right fist winding to the upper right, counterclockwise 270 degrees, around the shoulder circle.

The waist circle turns slightly left, the right fist half opens with its back gradually turning to face left and opening into an open palm with the qi ball in the palm fitting into the shoulder circle. Meanwhile, the left palm closes into a fist, falling with smooth rotation with its back facing up, then stretches open with the ball in the palm fitting into the hip circle.

The right hand turns outward clockwise with the elbow bending and drawing back to the cross center in front of the chest. The force lu wraps around the right arm through the outside and diffuses to the left hand through the back, left shoulder, and back of the left arm, triggering the left hand to turn outward counterclockwise, with the force exerting to the lower front from the root of the middle finger.

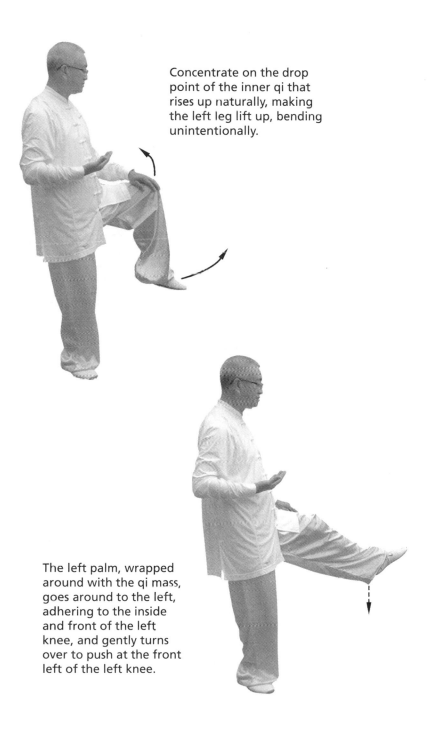

Concentrate on the drop point of the inner qi that rises up naturally, making the left leg lift up, bending unintentionally.

The left palm, wrapped around with the qi mass, goes around to the left, adhering to the inside and front of the left knee, and gently turns over to push at the front left of the left knee.

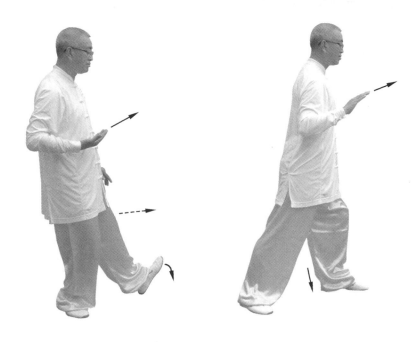

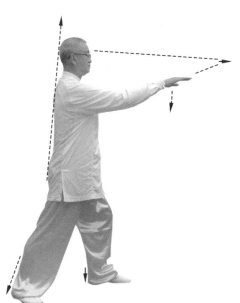

The left leg naturally falls down to a bow stance along with the inner qi fanning out; form a vertical san guan, with the inner qi triggered from the source of force, making the right arm reach forward along the shoulder circle, exerting an, peng, and ji through the root of the middle finger. The eyes look forward.

Right Brush Knee and Twist Step

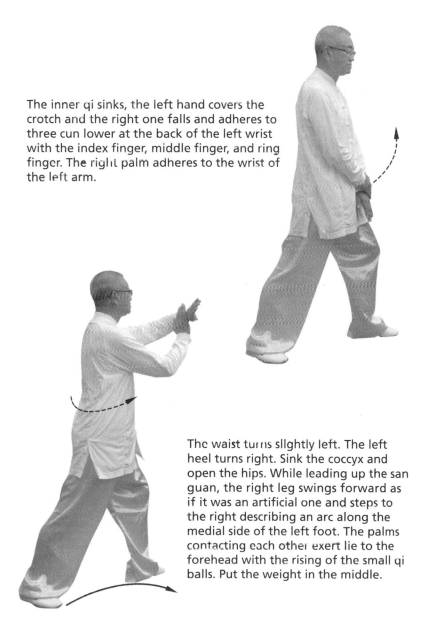

The inner qi sinks, the left hand covers the crotch and the right one falls and adheres to three cun lower at the back of the left wrist with the index finger, middle finger, and ring finger. The right palm adheres to the wrist of the left arm.

The waist turns slightly left. The left heel turns right. Sink the coccyx and open the hips. While leading up the san guan, the right leg swings forward as if it was an artificial one and steps to the right describing an arc along the medial side of the left foot. The palms contacting each other exert lie to the forehead with the rising of the small qi balls. Put the weight in the middle.

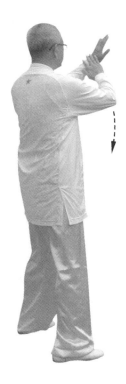

The palms fall to the front
of the crotch along the
vertical line of the cross
center in front of the chest,
following the falling ball.

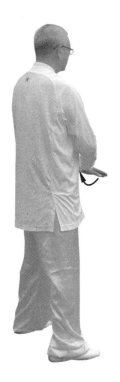

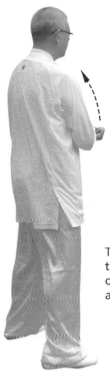

The left palm closes into a fist and turns inward with the back facing outward. The right one turns to adhere to the inside of the left wrist.

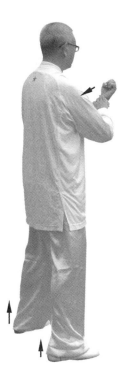

The left fist and right palm in contact exert peng up with the bouncing back of the inner qi from the ground. Bend the elbow with the balls of feet leaving the ground, the left fist draws back to the cross center in front of the chest, making the torso and the hands draw toward each other as if closing.

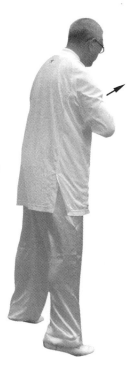

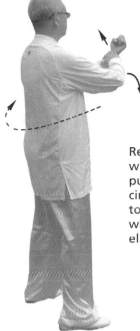

Resume the serenity of the mind, with the inner qi fanning outward, pushing the left fist to the shoulder circle. With the inner qi make the torso and hand repel as if opening, while retreating and bending the elbow.

The waist circle turns right briskly then left. Sink the shoulders and elbows, with the right fist winding toward the upper left, counterclockwise drawing a vertical circle on the shoulder circle for 270 degrees.

The waist circle turns slightly right, and the left fist slightly relaxes with its medial side turning left gradually and opening into a palm fitting the qi ball in the palm into the shoulder circle. Meanwhile, the right palm closes into a half-tightened fist falling with smooth rotation and the medial side facing down, then stretches open with the ball in the palm fitting into the hip circle.

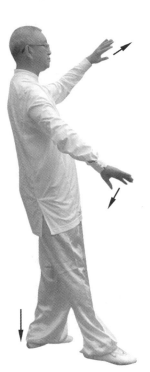

The left hand turns outward counterclockwise with the elbow bending and drawing into the cross center in front of the chest. The force lu diffuses to the right hand through the left arm, shoulders, back, and the right arm, triggering the right hand to turn outward counterclockwise, which exerts to the lower front from the root of the middle finger.

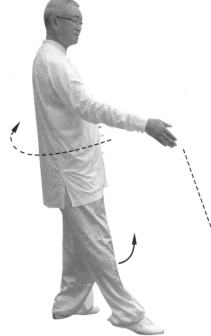

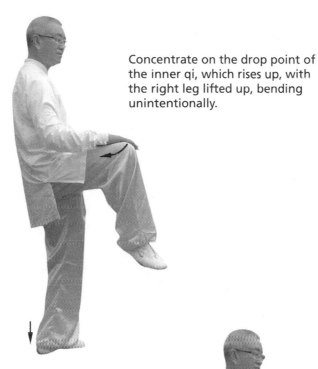

Concentrate on the drop point of
the inner qi, which rises up, with
the right leg lifted up, bending
unintentionally.

The right palm wrapped around
with the qi mass gradually
rotates inward, winding to the
left along the medial side and
the front of the right knee, and
pushes down to the front right
of the hip circle.

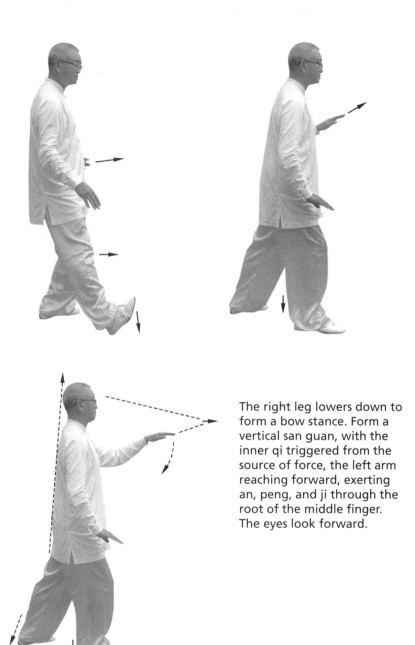

The right leg lowers down to form a bow stance. Form a vertical san guan, with the inner qi triggered from the source of force, the left arm reaching forward, exerting an, peng, and ji through the root of the middle finger. The eyes look forward.

Left Brush Knee and Twist Step

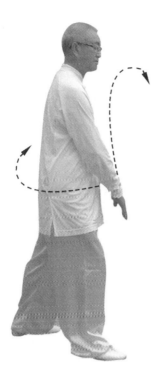

The right hand lifts to cover the crotch, with the left hand adhering to the back of the right wrist about three cun lower than the right wrist. Adhere with the index finger, middle finger, and ring finger. This is called contacting the palms.

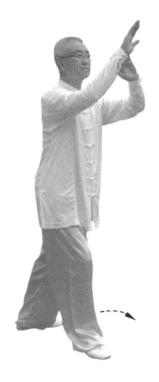

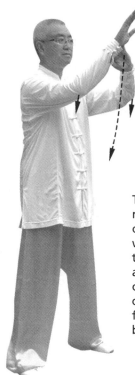

The waist slightly turns right, and the right heel turns right. Relax the coccyx, open the hips, and lead up the san guan with the left leg swinging forward toward the right leg as if it were an artificial leg and step to the left along the medial side of the right foot in an arc. The palms contacting each other exert lie to the forehead following the rising of the qi ball. Put your weight in the center.

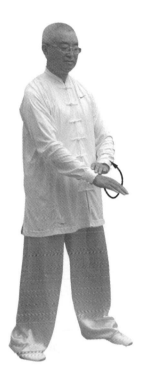

The palms in contact fall to the front of the crotch along the vertical line of the cross in front of the chest. They follow the falling of the balls of qi. The right palm closes into a fist and turns inward with the back of the fist facing outward, and the left hand turns to be close to the inside of the right wrist.

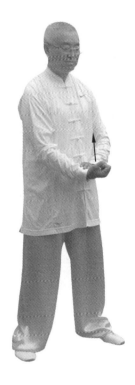

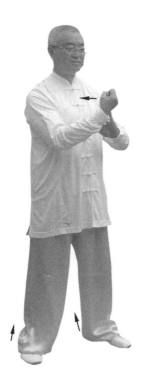

The right fist and left palm peng upward, following the bouncing back of the inner qi from the floor. Bend the elbow and move forward with the balls of the feet leaving the ground. The right fist at the cross center in front of the chest. The hands draw toward each other as if closing.

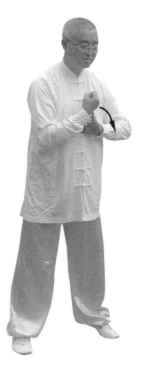

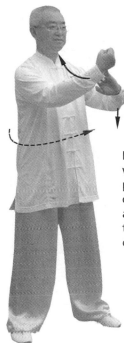

Resume the serenity of the mind, with the inner qi fanning outward, pushing the right fist to the shoulder circle. When straightening the elbow and retreating, the inner qi makes the torso and the hands repel each other as if they are about to open.

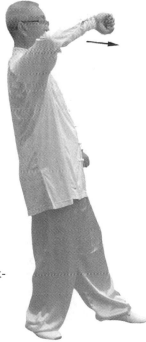

The waist circle turns left briskly then right. Relax the shoulders and sink the elbows with the right fist winding toward the upper right, moving counterclockwise 270 degrees around the shoulder circle.

The waist circle turns slightly left. The right fist half opens with its back gradually turning to face left and then the hand opens, with the qi ball in the palm fitting into the shoulder circle. Meanwhile, the left palm closes into a fist, falling with a smooth rotation with the back facing up. Then it stretches into an open hand with the ball in the palm fitting into the hip circle.

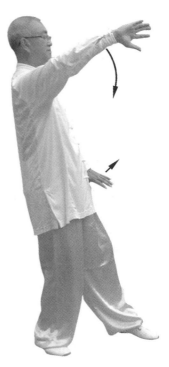

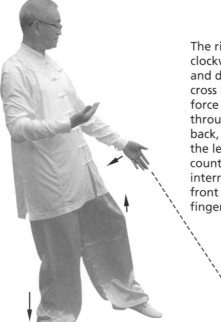

The right hand turns outward clockwise with the elbow bending and drawing into the center of the cross in front of the chest. The force lu diffuses to the right hand through the right arm, shoulders, back, and the right arm, triggering the left hand to turn outward counterclockwise. Then the internal force exerts to the lower front from the root of the middle finger.

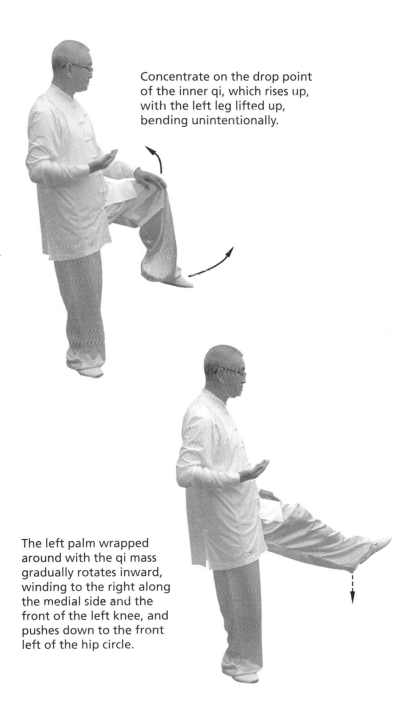

Concentrate on the drop point of the inner qi, which rises up, with the left leg lifted up, bending unintentionally.

The left palm wrapped around with the qi mass gradually rotates inward, winding to the right along the medial side and the front of the left knee, and pushes down to the front left of the hip circle.

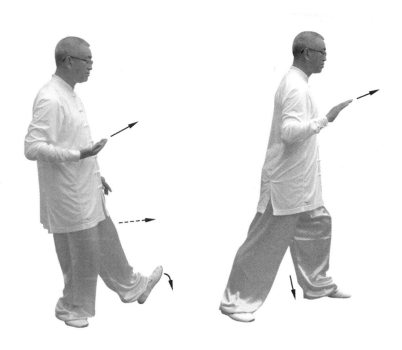

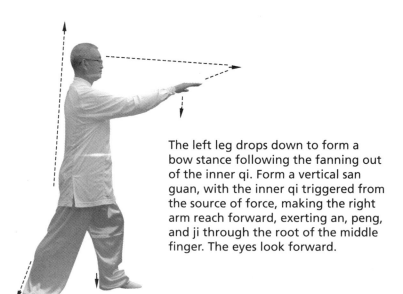

The left leg drops down to form a bow stance following the fanning out of the inner qi. Form a vertical san guan, with the inner qi triggered from the source of force, making the right arm reach forward, exerting an, peng, and ji through the root of the middle finger. The eyes look forward.

5. Strum the Lute

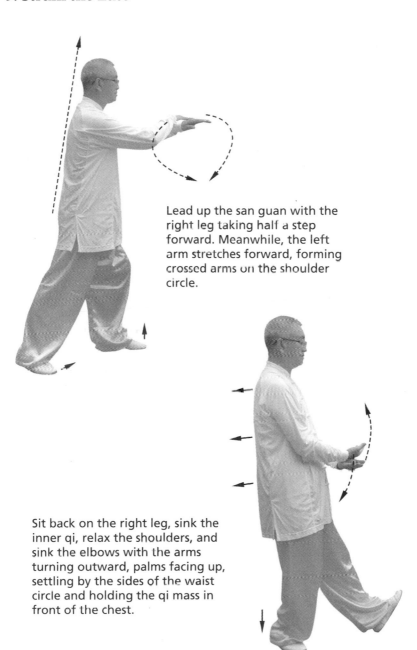

Lead up the san guan with the right leg taking half a step forward. Meanwhile, the left arm stretches forward, forming crossed arms on the shoulder circle.

Sit back on the right leg, sink the inner qi, relax the shoulders, and sink the elbows with the arms turning outward, palms facing up, settling by the sides of the waist circle and holding the qi mass in front of the chest.

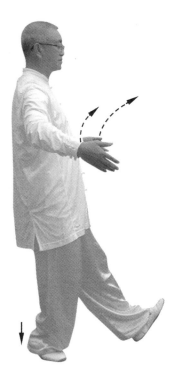

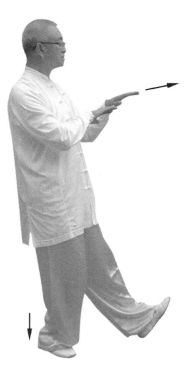

The palms move upward along the edge of the qi ball on both sides to the inner edge. Adhere to the qi ball and hold the mass with the palm with the left heel lifting up.

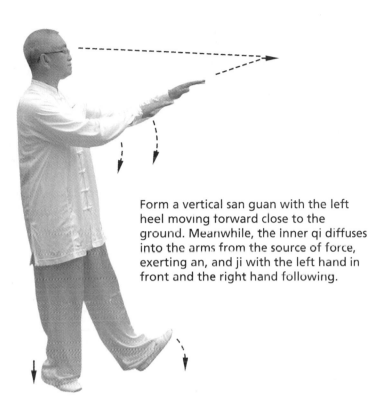

Form a vertical san guan with the left heel moving forward close to the ground. Meanwhile, the inner qi diffuses into the arms from the source of force, exerting an, and ji with the left hand in front and the right hand following.

6. Retreat and Repulse the Monkey

Left Retreat and Repulse the Monkey

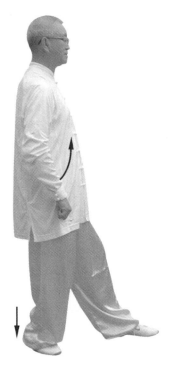

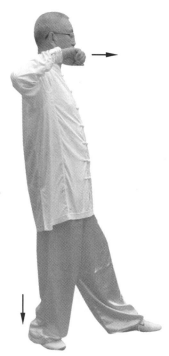

The inner qi sinks, the left foot drops to the ground, with the hands sinking into the hip circle and turning into half-grasped fists. The left fist stretches to form an open hand, the palm hanging on the left of the hip circles obliquely, with the right one rotating to the upper right, following the rising of the inner qi, opening into an open hand with the palm hanging on the right of the shoulder circle.

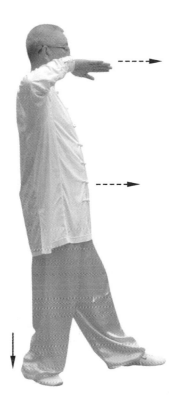

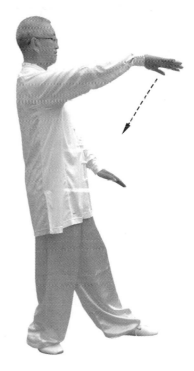

The palms post as if adhering to a piece of tilted glass, with the inner qi diffusing into the palms from the source of force, which reaches forward along the hip circle and shoulder circle.

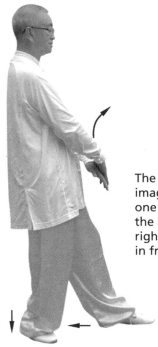

The left palm moves up along the imagined tilted glass, the right one moves downward. Then cover the back of the left hand with the right palm with the hands crossing in front of the abdomen.

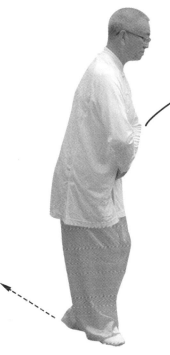

Resume the serenity of the mind, with a fine thread running through the san guan being pulled out backward from the coccyx, making the left leg naturally retreat, forming a retreating san guan and the right leg is forward, forming a bow stance. Meanwhile, the hands close into fists and lift to the front of the chest, following the inward twisting of the arms, with left fist inside and right one, crossing wrists. The inner qi penetrates to the front of the chest. The crossing fists exert peng to the shoulder circle, forming a leaning-forward san guan, with the eyes looking forward.

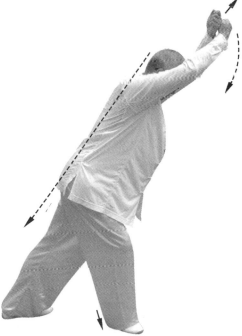

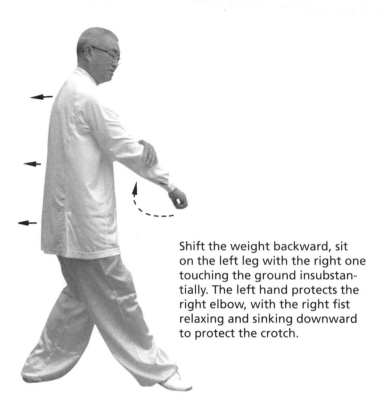

Shift the weight backward, sit on the left leg with the right one touching the ground insubstantially. The left hand protects the right elbow, with the right fist relaxing and sinking downward to protect the crotch.

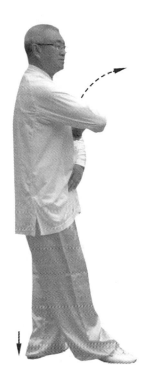

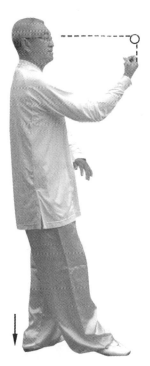

The right fist turns over and exerts peng forward with the root of the middle finger pointing ahead, to "approach the stars" posture.

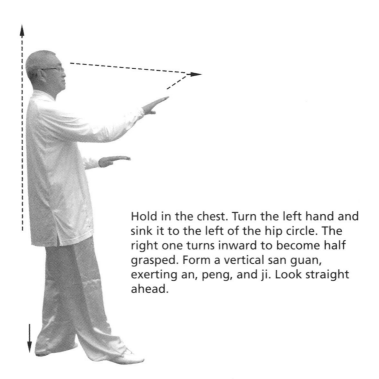

Hold in the chest. Turn the left hand and sink it to the left of the hip circle. The right one turns inward to become half grasped. Form a vertical san guan, exerting an, peng, and ji. Look straight ahead.

Right Retreat and Repulse the Monkey

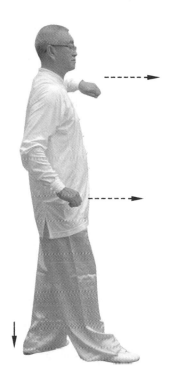

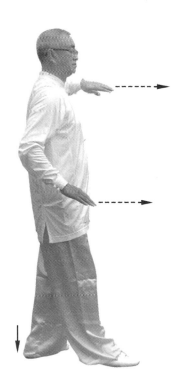

The inner qi sinks, the left foot falls to the ground, with the hands sinking into the hip circle and turning into half-grasped fists. The left fist stretches into a palm, turned outward 45 degrees, hanging on the left of the hip circles obliquely, with the right one rotating to the upper right following the rising of the inner qi, opening into a palm, turned outward 45 degrees, hanging on the right of the shoulder circle.

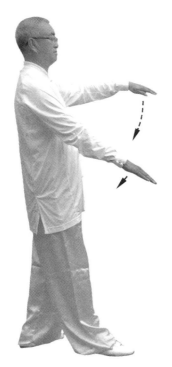

The palms post as if adhering to a piece of tilted glass, with the inner qi diffusing into the palms from the source of force, which reaches forward along the hip circle and shoulder circle.

The right palm moves up along the tilted glass; the left one moves downward. Then cover the back of the right hand with the left palm with the hands crossing in front of the abdomen.

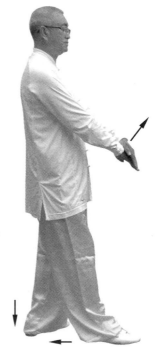

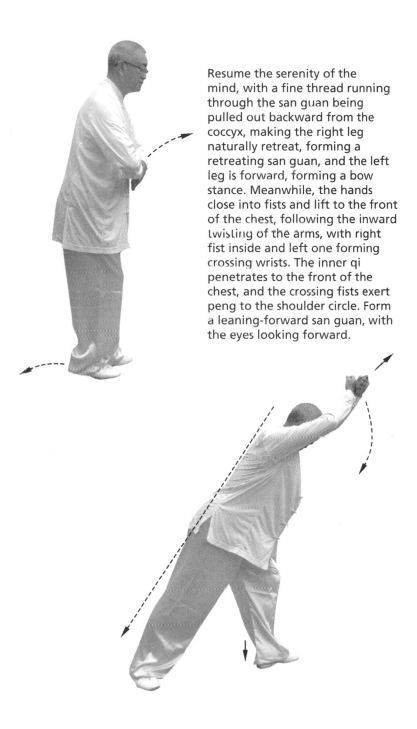

Resume the serenity of the mind, with a fine thread running through the san guan being pulled out backward from the coccyx, making the right leg naturally retreat, forming a retreating san guan, and the left leg is forward, forming a bow stance. Meanwhile, the hands close into fists and lift to the front of the chest, following the inward twisting of the arms, with right fist inside and left one forming crossing wrists. The inner qi penetrates to the front of the chest, and the crossing fists exert peng to the shoulder circle. Form a leaning-forward san guan, with the eyes looking forward.

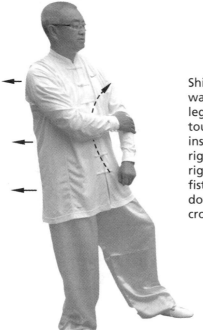

Shift the weight backward, sit on the right leg with the left one touching the ground insubstantially. The right hand protects the right elbow, with the left fist relaxing and sinking downward to protect the crotch.

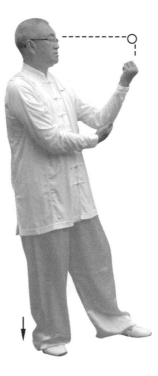

The left fist turns over and exerts peng forward with the root of the middle finger pointing ahead, to form the "approach the stars" posture.

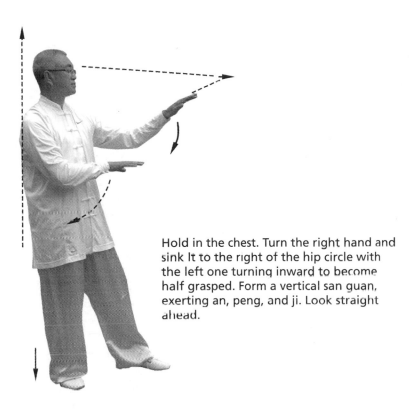

Hold in the chest. Turn the right hand and sink It to the right of the hip circle with the left one turning inward to become half grasped. Form a vertical san guan, exerting an, peng, and ji. Look straight ahead.

(Repeat "Retreat and Repulse the Monkey.")

7. Left and Right Grasp the Peacock's Tail

Left Grasp the Peacock's Tail

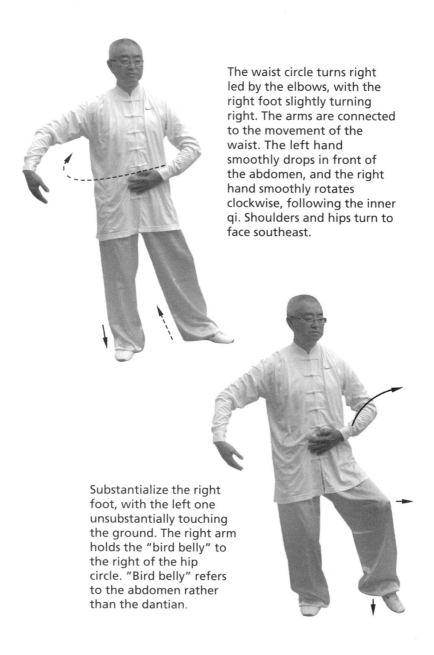

The waist circle turns right led by the elbows, with the right foot slightly turning right. The arms are connected to the movement of the waist. The left hand smoothly drops in front of the abdomen, and the right hand smoothly rotates clockwise, following the inner qi. Shoulders and hips turn to face southeast.

Substantialize the right foot, with the left one unsubstantially touching the ground. The right arm holds the "bird belly" to the right of the hip circle. "Bird belly" refers to the abdomen rather than the dantian.

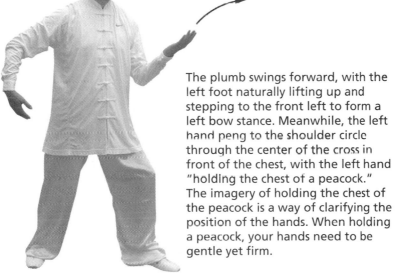

The plumb swings forward, with the left foot naturally lifting up and stepping to the front left to form a left bow stance. Meanwhile, the left hand peng to the shoulder circle through the center of the cross in front of the chest, with the left hand "holding the chest of a peacock." The imagery of holding the chest of the peacock is a way of clarifying the position of the hands. When holding a peacock, your hands need to be gentle yet firm.

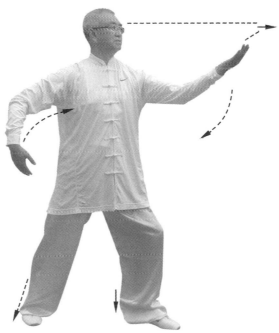

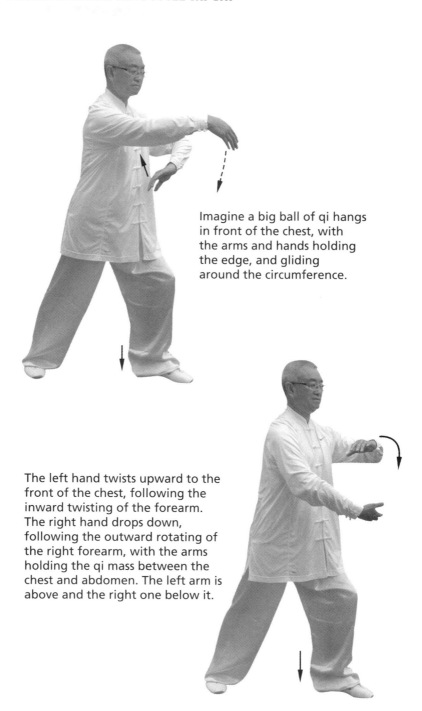

Imagine a big ball of qi hangs
in front of the chest, with
the arms and hands holding
the edge, and gliding
around the circumference.

The left hand twists upward to the
front of the chest, following the
inward twisting of the forearm.
The right hand drops down,
following the outward rotating of
the right forearm, with the arms
holding the qi mass between the
chest and abdomen. The left arm is
above and the right one below it.

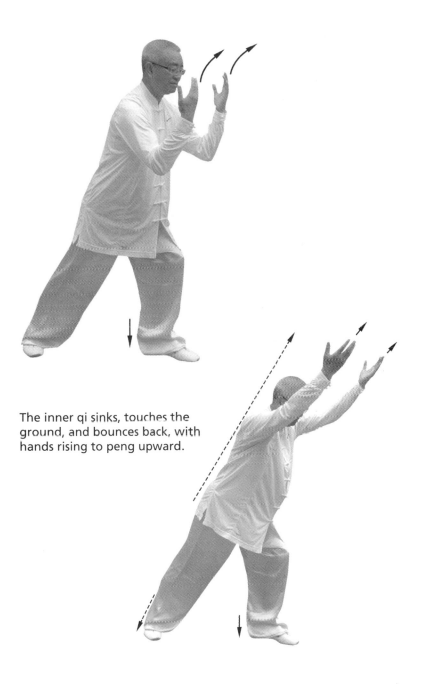

The inner qi sinks, touches the ground, and bounces back, with hands rising to peng upward.

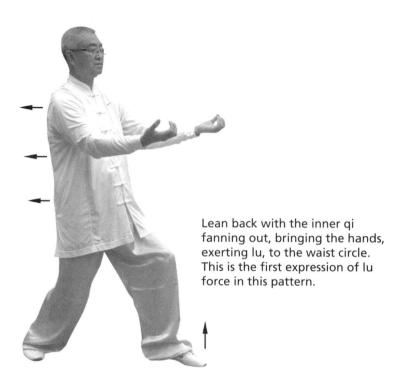

Lean back with the inner qi fanning out, bringing the hands, exerting lu, to the waist circle. This is the first expression of lu force in this pattern.

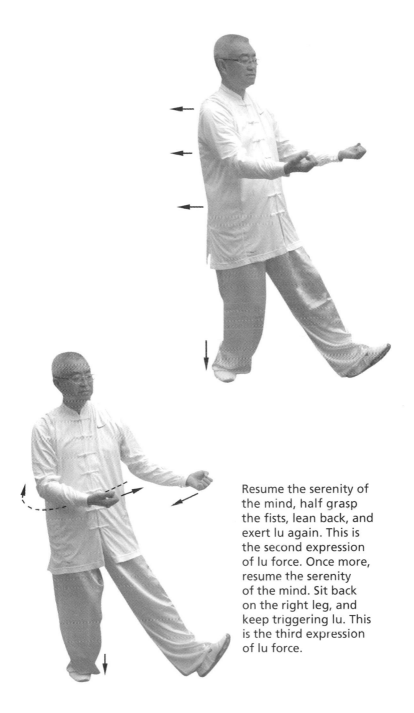

Resume the serenity of the mind, half grasp the fists, lean back, and exert lu again. This is the second expression of lu force. Once more, resume the serenity of the mind. Sit back on the right leg, and keep triggering lu. This is the third expression of lu force.

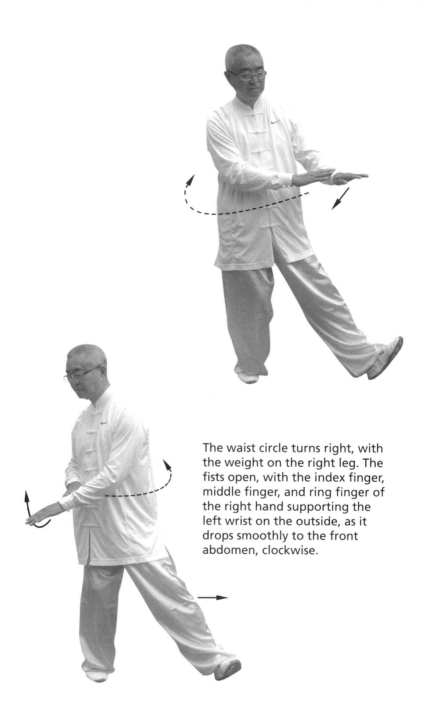

The waist circle turns right, with the weight on the right leg. The fists open, with the index finger, middle finger, and ring finger of the right hand supporting the left wrist on the outside, as it drops smoothly to the front abdomen, clockwise.

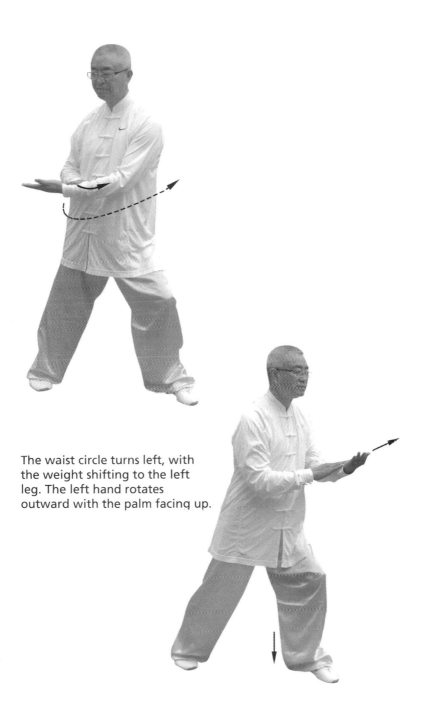

The waist circle turns left, with the weight shifting to the left leg. The left hand rotates outward with the palm facing up.

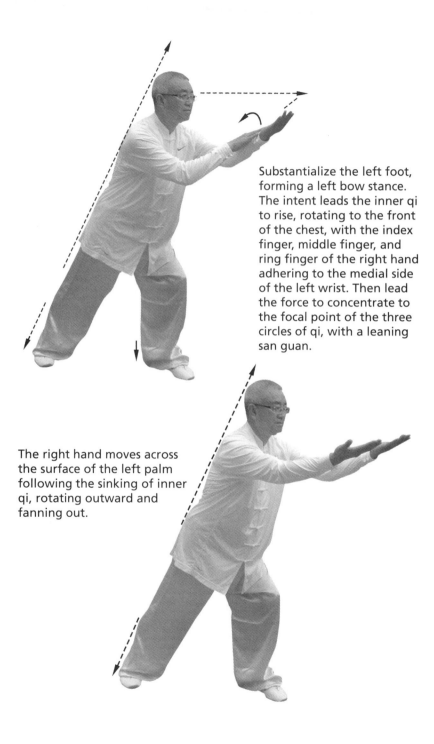

Substantialize the left foot, forming a left bow stance. The intent leads the inner qi to rise, rotating to the front of the chest, with the index finger, middle finger, and ring finger of the right hand adhering to the medial side of the left wrist. Then lead the force to concentrate to the focal point of the three circles of qi, with a leaning san guan.

The right hand moves across the surface of the left palm following the sinking of inner qi, rotating outward and fanning out.

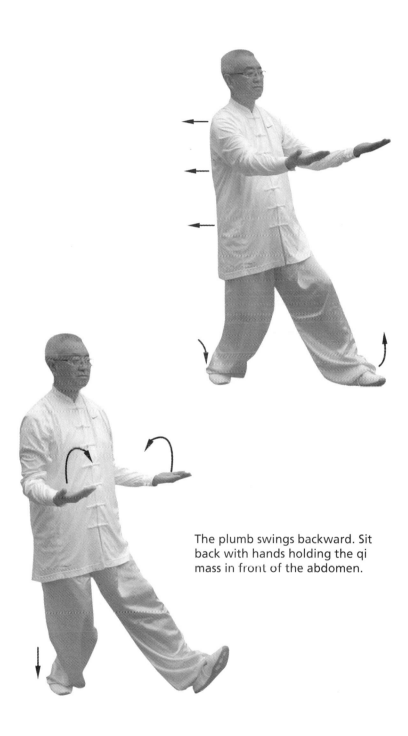

The plumb swings backward. Sit back with hands holding the qi mass in front of the abdomen.

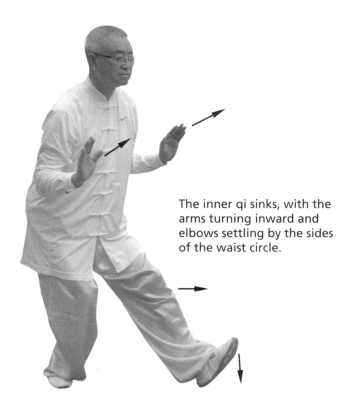

The inner qi sinks, with the arms turning inward and elbows settling by the sides of the waist circle.

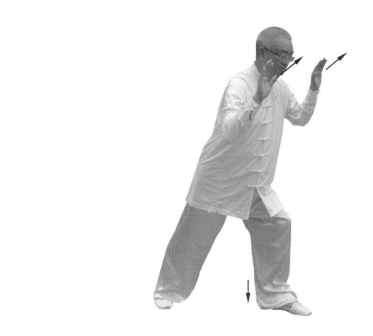

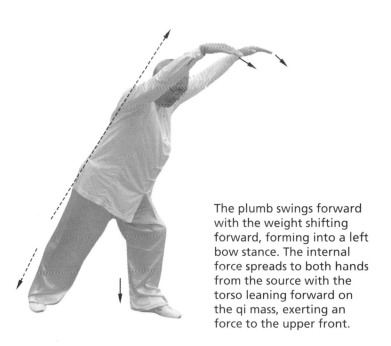

The plumb swings forward with the weight shifting forward, forming into a left bow stance. The internal force spreads to both hands from the source with the torso leaning forward on the qi mass, exerting an force to the upper front.

Right Grasp the Peacock's Tail

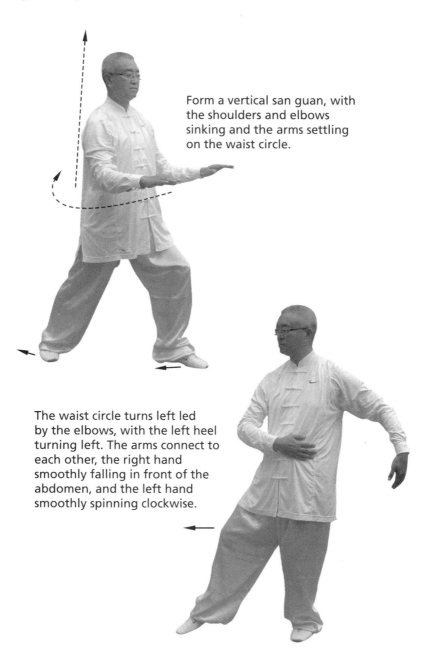

Form a vertical san guan, with the shoulders and elbows sinking and the arms settling on the waist circle.

The waist circle turns left led by the elbows, with the left heel turning left. The arms connect to each other, the right hand smoothly falling in front of the abdomen, and the left hand smoothly spinning clockwise.

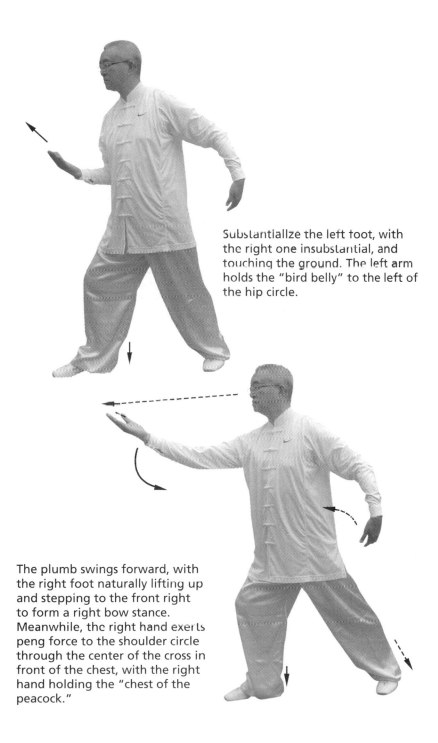

Substantialize the left foot, with the right one insubstantial, and touching the ground. The left arm holds the "bird belly" to the left of the hip circle.

The plumb swings forward, with the right foot naturally lifting up and stepping to the front right to form a right bow stance. Meanwhile, the right hand exerts peng force to the shoulder circle through the center of the cross in front of the chest, with the right hand holding the "chest of the peacock."

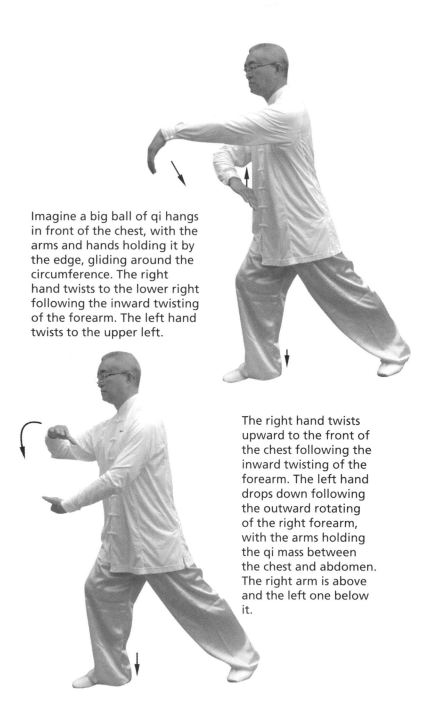

Imagine a big ball of qi hangs in front of the chest, with the arms and hands holding it by the edge, gliding around the circumference. The right hand twists to the lower right following the inward twisting of the forearm. The left hand twists to the upper left.

The right hand twists upward to the front of the chest following the inward twisting of the forearm. The left hand drops down following the outward rotating of the right forearm, with the arms holding the qi mass between the chest and abdomen. The right arm is above and the left one below it.

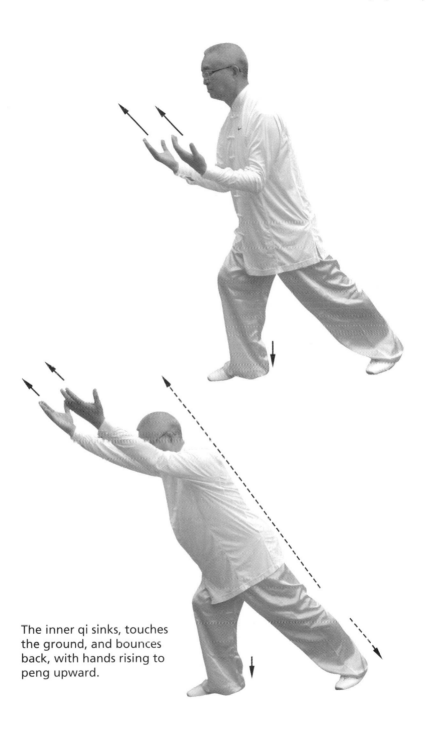

The inner qi sinks, touches the ground, and bounces back, with hands rising to peng upward.

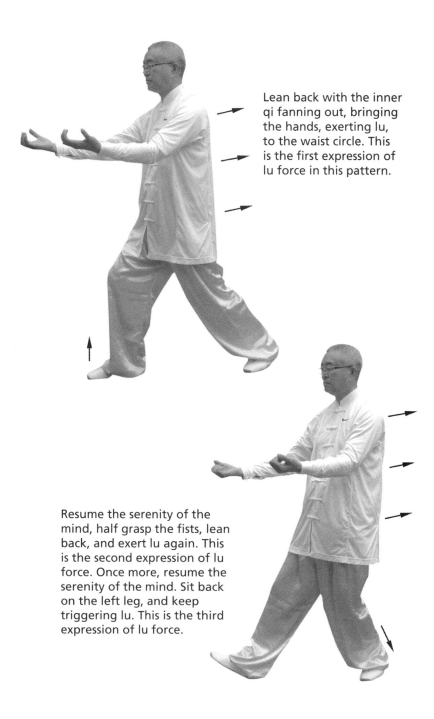

Lean back with the inner qi fanning out, bringing the hands, exerting lu, to the waist circle. This is the first expression of lu force in this pattern.

Resume the serenity of the mind, half grasp the fists, lean back, and exert lu again. This is the second expression of lu force. Once more, resume the serenity of the mind. Sit back on the left leg, and keep triggering lu. This is the third expression of lu force.

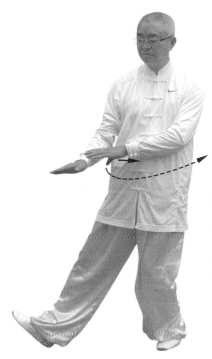

The waist circle turns left, the fists open, with the index finger, middle finger, and ring finger of the left hand supporting the right wrist on the outside, as they fall smoothly clockwise to the front abdomen.

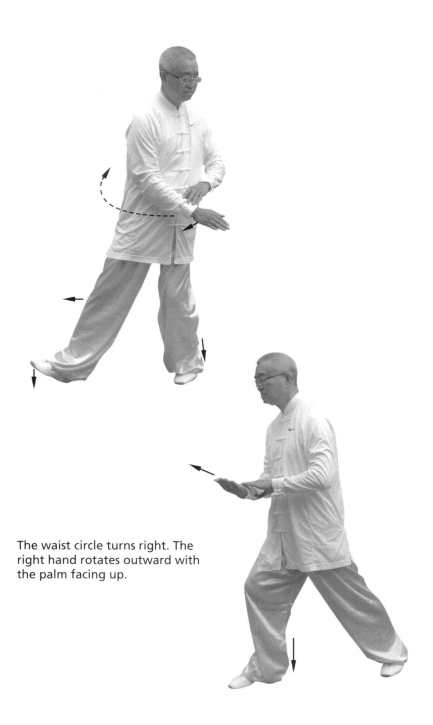

The waist circle turns right. The right hand rotates outward with the palm facing up.

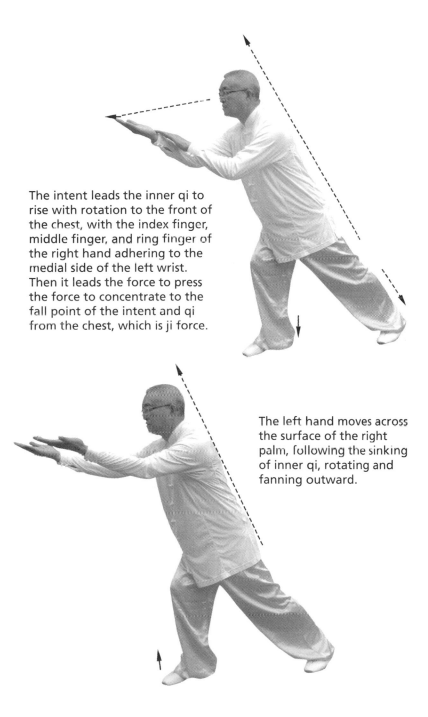

The intent leads the inner qi to rise with rotation to the front of the chest, with the index finger, middle finger, and ring finger of the right hand adhering to the medial side of the left wrist. Then it leads the force to press the force to concentrate to the fall point of the intent and qi from the chest, which is ji force.

The left hand moves across the surface of the right palm, following the sinking of inner qi, rotating and fanning outward.

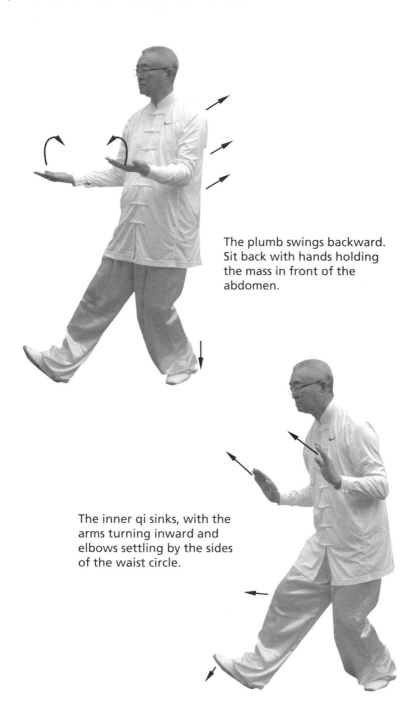

The plumb swings backward. Sit back with hands holding the mass in front of the abdomen.

The inner qi sinks, with the arms turning inward and elbows settling by the sides of the waist circle.

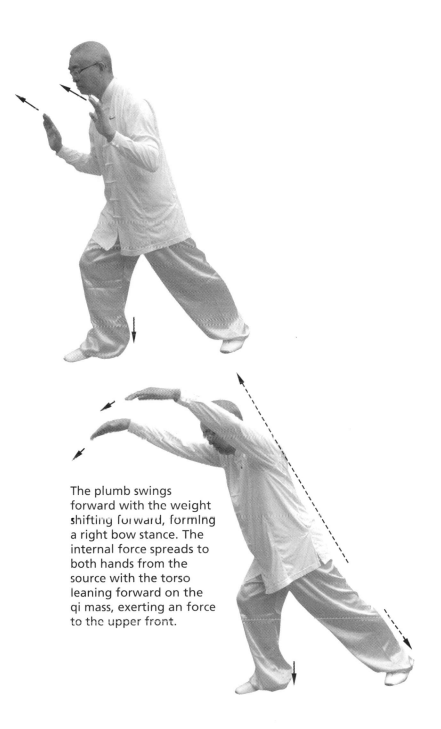

The plumb swings forward with the weight shifting forward, forming a right bow stance. The internal force spreads to both hands from the source with the torso leaning forward on the qi mass, exerting an force to the upper front.

8. Cloud Hands

First Open and Close Cloud Hands

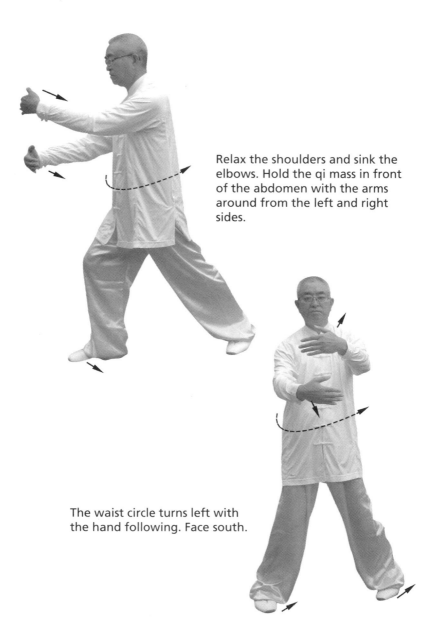

Relax the shoulders and sink the elbows. Hold the qi mass in front of the abdomen with the arms around from the left and right sides.

The waist circle turns left with the hand following. Face south.

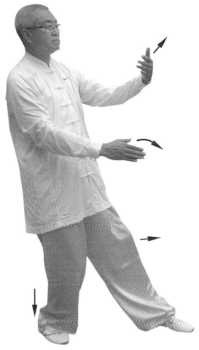

The waist circle keeps turning left, with the right toes turning inward and the hands following. Face southeast. The weight roots on the right foot, with the left foot on the ground, exerting cai force. The left hand slides and pushes downward to the left of the hip circle describing half a dome. The right hand draws up through the chest and turns into a fist along the other half dome.

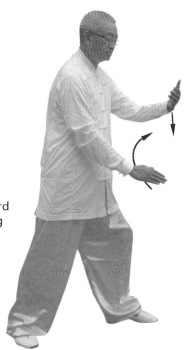

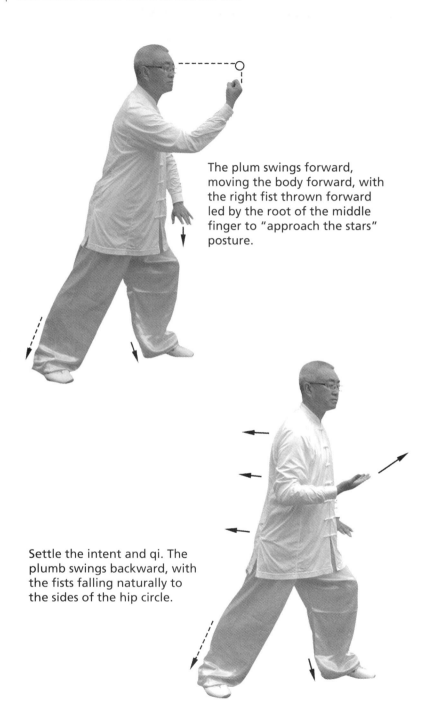

The plum swings forward, moving the body forward, with the right fist thrown forward led by the root of the middle finger to "approach the stars" posture.

Settle the intent and qi. The plumb swings backward, with the fists falling naturally to the sides of the hip circle.

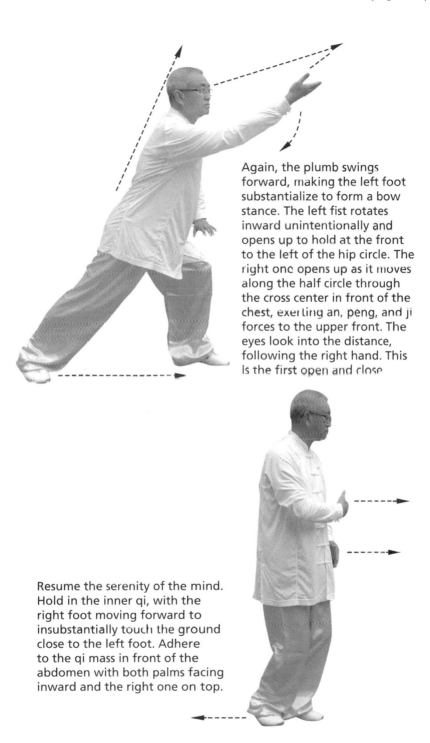

Again, the plumb swings forward, making the left foot substantialize to form a bow stance. The left fist rotates inward unintentionally and opens up to hold at the front to the left of the hip circle. The right one opens up as it moves along the half circle through the cross center in front of the chest, exerting an, peng, and ji forces to the upper front. The eyes look into the distance, following the right hand. This is the first open and close

Resume the serenity of the mind. Hold in the inner qi, with the right foot moving forward to insubstantially touch the ground close to the left foot. Adhere to the qi mass in front of the abdomen with both palms facing inward and the right one on top.

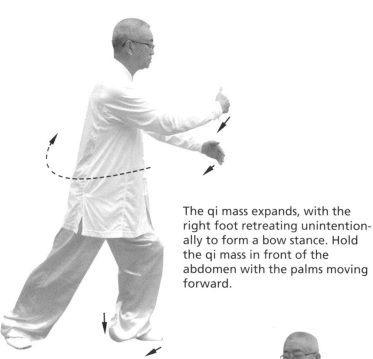

The qi mass expands, with the right foot retreating unintentionally to form a bow stance. Hold the qi mass in front of the abdomen with the palms moving forward.

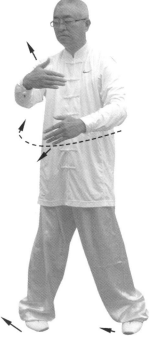

The waist circle turns right. The hands move right along with the torso, with the right one exerting lie force. The left one exerts cai force. Face southwest. This is right cloud hands.

Second Open and Close Cloud Hands

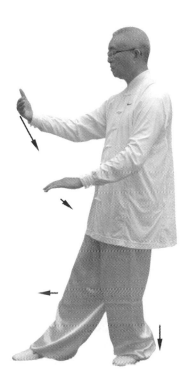

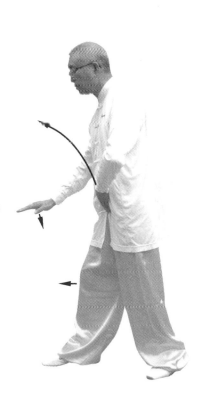

The weight roots on the left foot, with the right foot stepping down, exerting cai force. The right hand slides along a half circle to the right side, exerting an force to the right hip circle, with the left hand becoming a fist drawing up along a half circle through the chest.

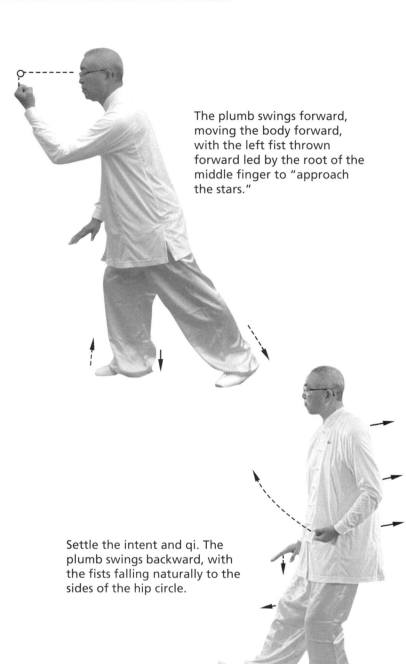

The plumb swings forward, moving the body forward, with the left fist thrown forward led by the root of the middle finger to "approach the stars."

Settle the intent and qi. The plumb swings backward, with the fists falling naturally to the sides of the hip circle.

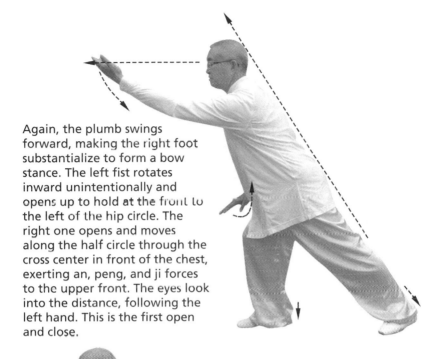

Again, the plumb swings forward, making the right foot substantialize to form a bow stance. The left fist rotates inward unintentionally and opens up to hold at the front to the left of the hip circle. The right one opens and moves along the half circle through the cross center in front of the chest, exerting an, peng, and ji forces to the upper front. The eyes look into the distance, following the left hand. This is the first open and close.

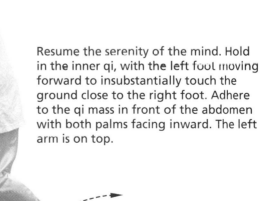

Resume the serenity of the mind. Hold in the inner qi, with the left foot moving forward to insubstantially touch the ground close to the right foot. Adhere to the qi mass in front of the abdomen with both palms facing inward. The left arm is on top.

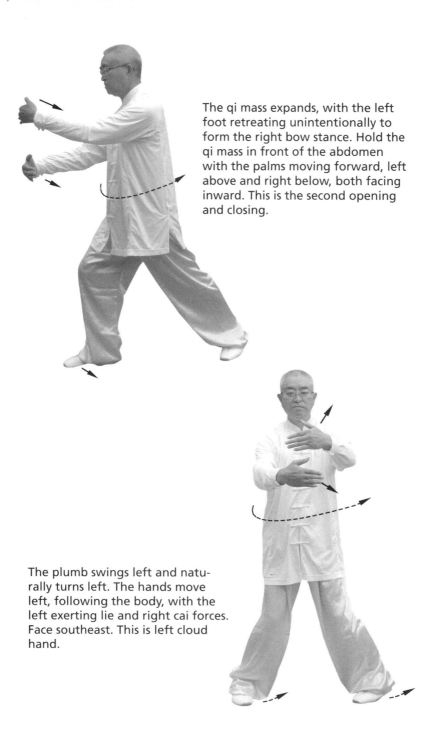

The qi mass expands, with the left foot retreating unintentionally to form the right bow stance. Hold the qi mass in front of the abdomen with the palms moving forward, left above and right below, both facing inward. This is the second opening and closing.

The plumb swings left and naturally turns left. The hands move left, following the body, with the left exerting lie and right cai forces. Face southeast. This is left cloud hand.

Third Open and Close Cloud Hands

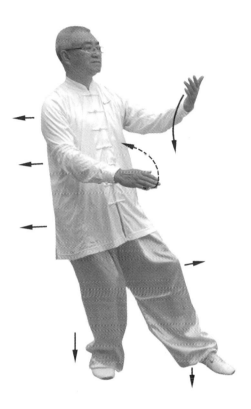

The weight roots on the right foot, with the left foot on the ground, exerting cai force. The left hand slides and pushes down to the left of the hip circle, describing half a dome. The right hand draws up in front of the chest and turns into a fist along the other half dome.

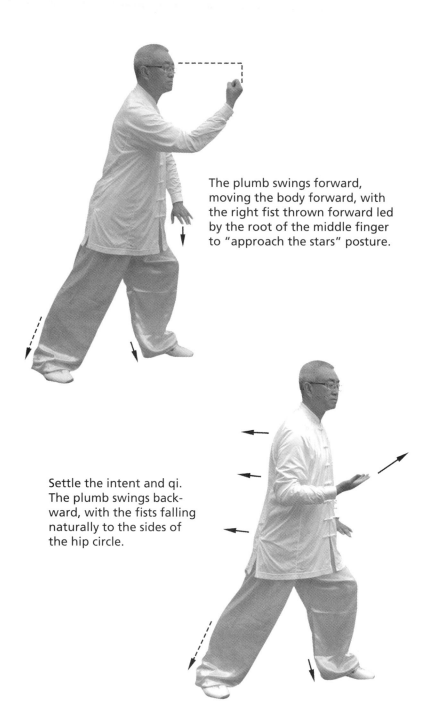

The plumb swings forward, moving the body forward, with the right fist thrown forward led by the root of the middle finger to "approach the stars" posture.

Settle the intent and qi. The plumb swings backward, with the fists falling naturally to the sides of the hip circle.

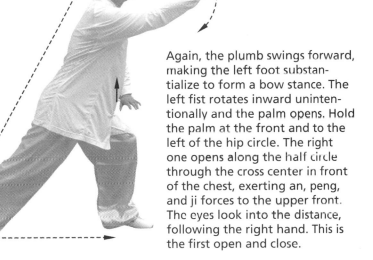

Again, the plumb swings forward, making the left foot substantialize to form a bow stance. The left fist rotates inward unintentionally and the palm opens. Hold the palm at the front and to the left of the hip circle. The right one opens along the half circle through the cross center in front of the chest, exerting an, peng, and ji forces to the upper front. The eyes look into the distance, following the right hand. This is the first open and close.

Resume the serenity of the mind, and hold in the inner qi. The right foot moves forward, insubstantially touching the ground close to the left foot. Adhere to the qi mass in front of the abdomen with both palms facing inward. The right one is on top.

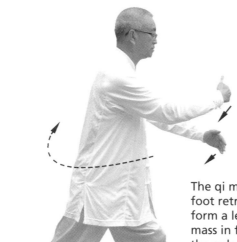

The qi mass expands, with the right foot retreating unintentionally to form a left bow stance. Hold the mass in front of the abdomen while the palms move forward, right above and left below, both facing inward. This is the second opening and closing of the third open and close cloud hands.

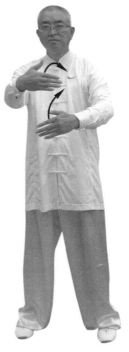

The plumb swings right and naturally turns right. The hands move right, following the body, with the right exerting lie force and the left exerting cai force. Face south with weight in the middle. Turn the hands inward, forming the shape of a "dragon mouth." Imagine swallowing the ball in front of the chest to the back, which is called "dragon swallowing pearl." This is the last closing of the third open and close cloud hands.

The ball of intent and qi is spit out from the back of the hands shooting through the "dragon mouth" formed by the hands. The hands open and expand influenced by the qi ball, which is called "dragon spitting pearl." This is the last opening of the third open and close cloud hands.

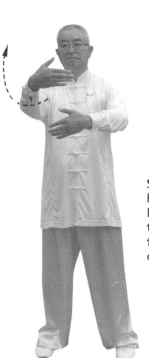

Settle the intent and qi. The right hand rotates outward clockwise. The left hand rotates slightly inward, with the palms facing inward. The inner qi fans out, making the palm extend outward, exerting peng force.

9. Single Whip

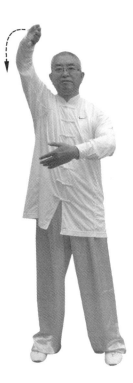

The inner qi rotates and rises, making the right hand rotate counterclockwise, with the palm facing right, exerting peng force up to the forehead along the outer circle of the crescent.

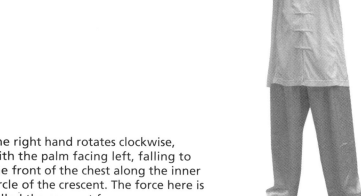

The right hand rotates clockwise, with the palm facing left, falling to the front of the chest along the inner circle of the crescent. The force here is called the crescent force.

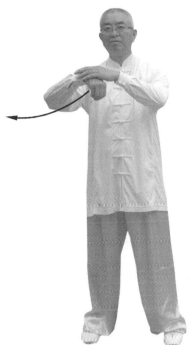

The left palm holds the back of the right hand, rotating inward to the cross center in front of the chest along with the inner qi holding inward in the chest. The fingers of the right hand gather to form a hook with the wrist rotating inward till the tip of the hook points downward. Place the index finger, middle finger, and ring finger of the left hand at the top of the right wrist to support it.

The right forearm rolls to the upper right from the right of the horizontal line of the cross, exerting the force of rolling. Think of the forearm as a rolling pin, the thick round bar used to roll out dough.

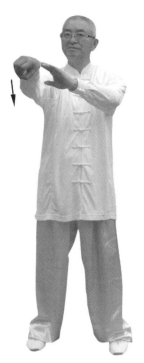

The right hook slightly rotates outward along with the forearm, with the force moving to the ulna front from the radius. The right arm led by the ulna rasps across to the front left, exerting a rasping force.

The right elbow sinks back down along with zhou force, diffusing at the elbow, exerting the force of folding to the back.

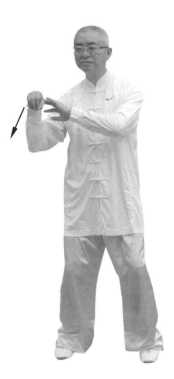

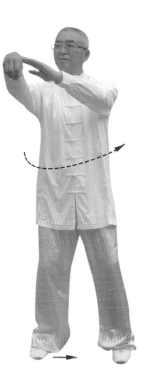

The force at the elbow flows to the wrist through the forearm, with the hook tip hanging down, exerting the force of folding to the front.

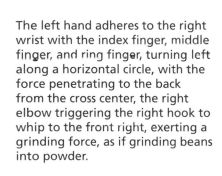

The left hand adheres to the right wrist with the index finger, middle finger, and ring finger, turning left along a horizontal circle, with the force penetrating to the back from the cross center, the right elbow triggering the right hook to whip to the front right, exerting a grinding force, as if grinding beans into powder.

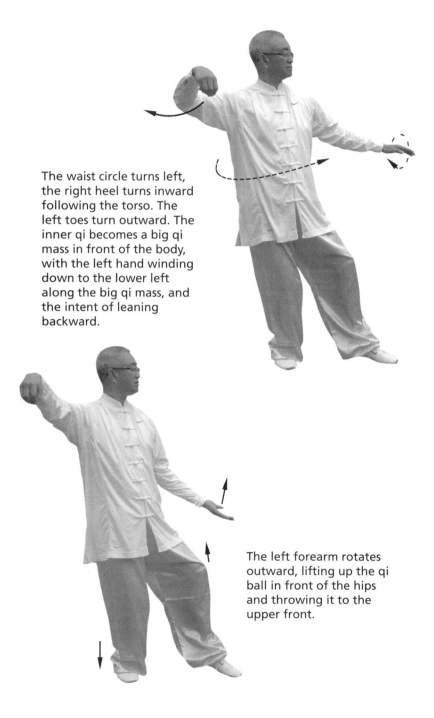

The waist circle turns left, the right heel turns inward following the torso. The left toes turn outward. The inner qi becomes a big qi mass in front of the body, with the left hand winding down to the lower left along the big qi mass, and the intent of leaning backward.

The left forearm rotates outward, lifting up the qi ball in front of the hips and throwing it to the upper front.

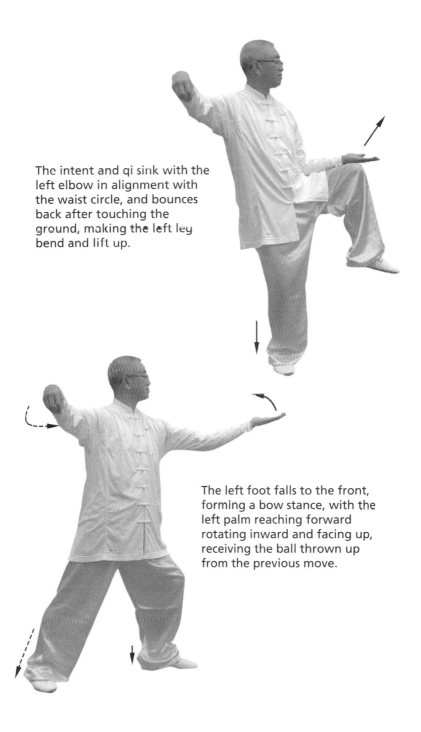

The intent and qi sink with the left elbow in alignment with the waist circle, and bounces back after touching the ground, making the left leg bend and lift up.

The left foot falls to the front, forming a bow stance, with the left palm reaching forward rotating inward and facing up, receiving the ball thrown up from the previous move.

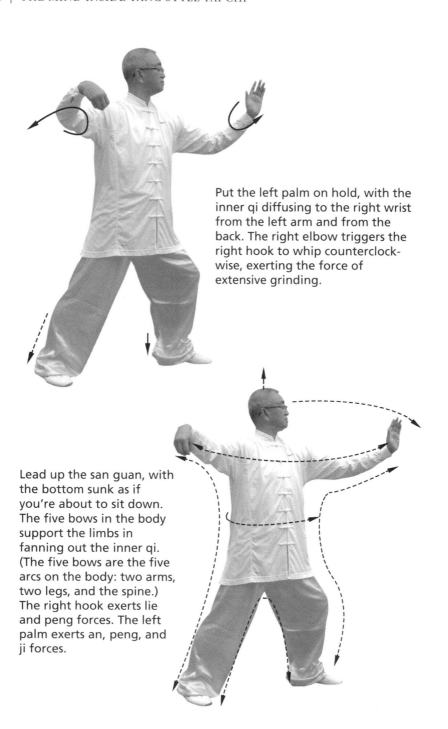

Put the left palm on hold, with the inner qi diffusing to the right wrist from the left arm and from the back. The right elbow triggers the right hook to whip counterclockwise, exerting the force of extensive grinding.

Lead up the san guan, with the bottom sunk as if you're about to sit down. The five bows in the body support the limbs in fanning out the inner qi. (The five bows are the five arcs on the body: two arms, two legs, and the spine.) The right hook exerts lie and peng forces. The left palm exerts an, peng, and ji forces.

10. High Pat on Horse

The waist circle turns left, with left rotation moving along the shoulder circle from the left palm. The right hook stretches to the side. The inner qi diffuses to the right hook from the left hand through the shoulder circle at the back, which is the inner qi moving along the shoulder circle.

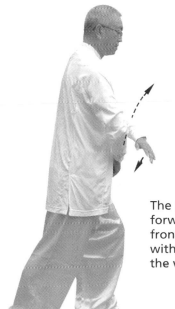

The right foot moves half a step forward. The right hook falls to the front of the crotch and becomes a fist, with the left arm held horizontal on the waist circle.

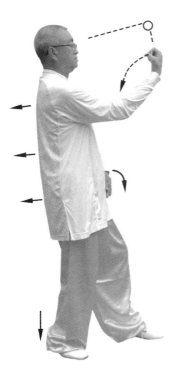

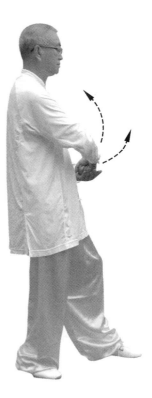

Lean back, triggering the inner qi to move around a vertical circle to the forehead through the back from the crotch. Meet the left palm with the right fist in front of the chest.

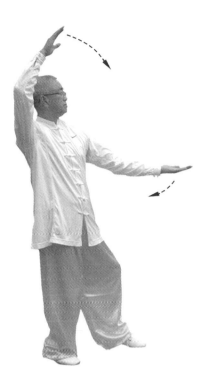

Substantialize the right foot, with the left foot insubstantially touching the ground and the right fist falling to the front of the abdomen following the inner qi. The left palm rotates, palm facing up, with the right fist falling on the left palm. This is how the inner qi moves along the vertical circle.

The inner qi goes up along a tilted circle to the front right of the shoulder circle through the back from the hip left, and meets with the right fist, which rotates inward and turns into an open palm with the rising of the inner qi and forms a link of qi with the left palm reaching forward and facing upward.

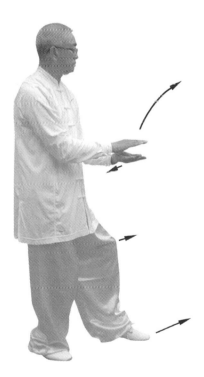

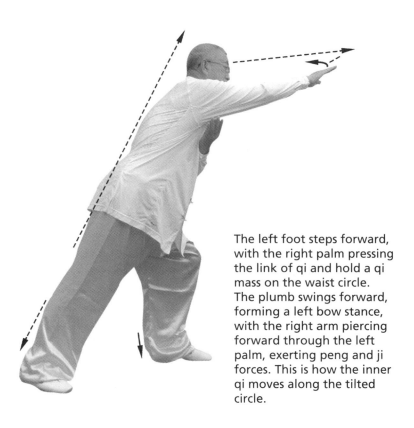

The left foot steps forward, with the right palm pressing the link of qi and hold a qi mass on the waist circle. The plumb swings forward, forming a left bow stance, with the right arm piercing forward through the left palm, exerting peng and ji forces. This is how the inner qi moves along the tilted circle.

11. Right Splitting Foot

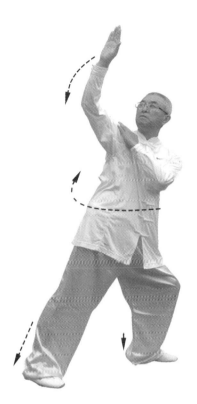

The waist circle briskly turns left then right. The feet are pigeon toed with the right foot insubstantially on the ground. The right hand rotates back clockwise from the front left to the back right, with the left hand turning and twisting right, gently protecting the right shoulder. The eyes follow the right hand.

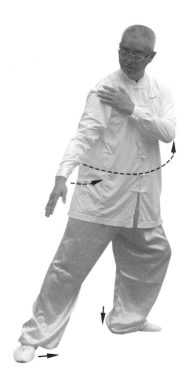

The left hand protects the right elbow. The right hand rotates inward, following the arm describing an upper left arc, protecting the left chest first, then the face, and then stretches to the upper front of the head.

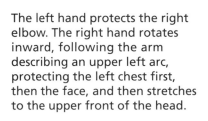

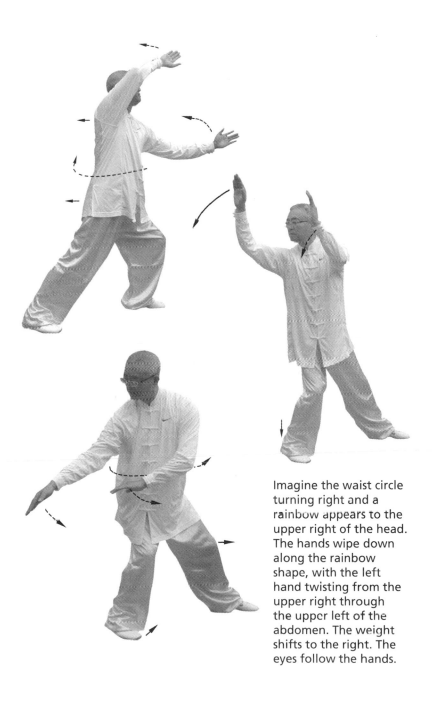

Imagine the waist circle turning right and a rainbow appears to the upper right of the head. The hands wipe down along the rainbow shape, with the left hand twisting from the upper right through the upper left of the abdomen. The weight shifts to the right. The eyes follow the hands.

The weight moves to the left, following the left lu force of both hands. The waist circle turns left, with the left ball of the foot turning outward, forming a left bow stance. The left arm goes around the hip circle and the arms naturally fall on the hip circle.

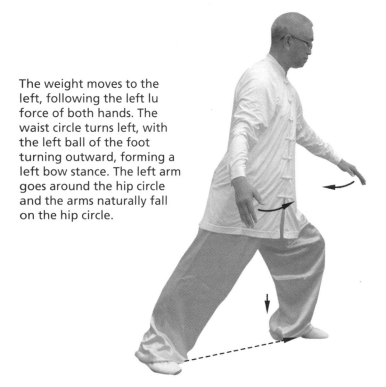

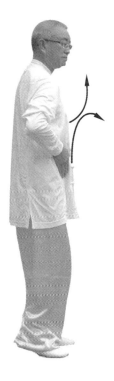

Form a substantial left leg and insubstantial right, with the hand moving upward close to the abdomen, then piercing and stretching to both sides separately when reaching the upper abdomen with the palms facing up. Face east.

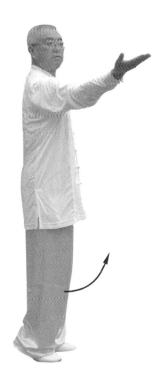

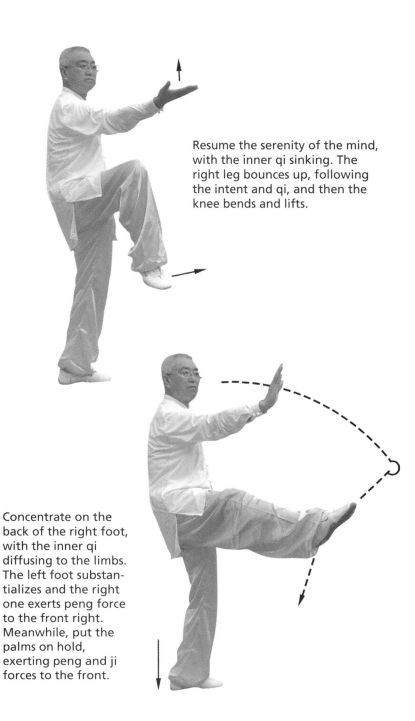

Resume the serenity of the mind, with the inner qi sinking. The right leg bounces up, following the intent and qi, and then the knee bends and lifts.

Concentrate on the back of the right foot, with the inner qi diffusing to the limbs. The left foot substantializes and the right one exerts peng force to the front right. Meanwhile, put the palms on hold, exerting peng and ji forces to the front.

12. Punch the Ears with Fists

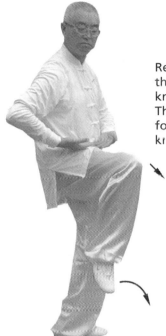

Resume the serenity of the mind, with the right leg bending and lifting the knee. The toes point downward. The hands rotate outward with cai force and fall to the sides of the right knee with the palms facing upward.

The inner qi sinks. The plumb swings forward, making the right foot fall to the front, forming a bow stance. The hands rotate inward while closing into fists, with the force flowing to the fists from the source of force.

The fists rotate upward to the front of the head, with the eyes of the fists facing downward, exerting peng and ji from the roots of the middle fingers through the backs of the fists. The eye of the fist is the space formed when the thumb, index finger close as part of making a fist.

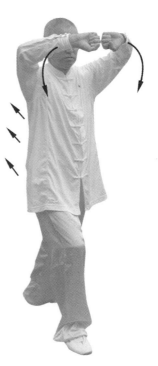

The fists draw back, exerting lu force, with the shoulders and hips facing southeast.

13. Left Kick

The weight is substantial on the right leg and insubstantial on the left, while the hands move upward close to the body from the lower abdomen.

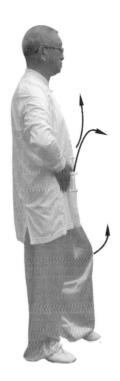

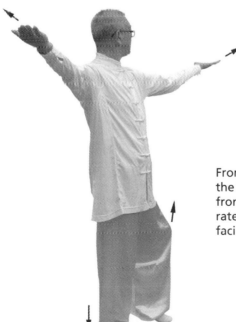

From the upper abdomen, the hands pierce to the front of both sides separately with the palms facing upward. Face east.

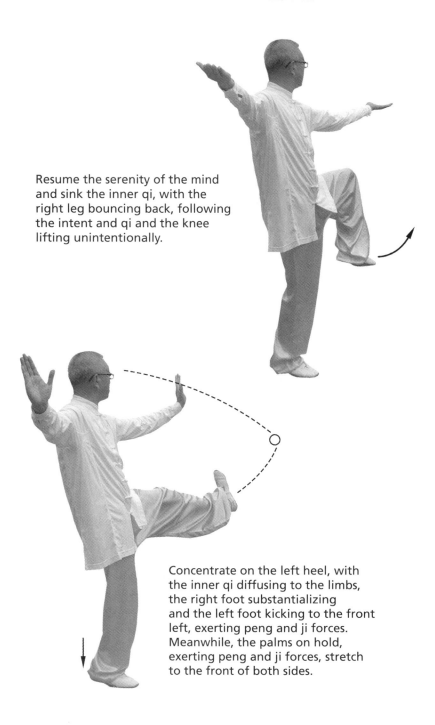

Resume the serenity of the mind and sink the inner qi, with the right leg bouncing back, following the intent and qi and the knee lifting unintentionally.

Concentrate on the left heel, with the inner qi diffusing to the limbs, the right foot substantializing and the left foot kicking to the front left, exerting peng and ji forces. Meanwhile, the palms on hold, exerting peng and ji forces, stretch to the front of both sides.

14. Left and Right Fair Lady Works the Shuttle

Left Fair Lady Works the Shuttle

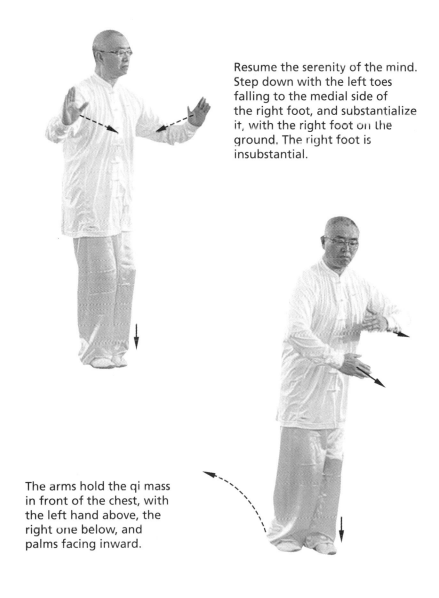

Resume the serenity of the mind. Step down with the left toes falling to the medial side of the right foot, and substantialize it, with the right foot on the ground. The right foot is insubstantial.

The arms hold the qi mass in front of the chest, with the left hand above, the right one below, and palms facing inward.

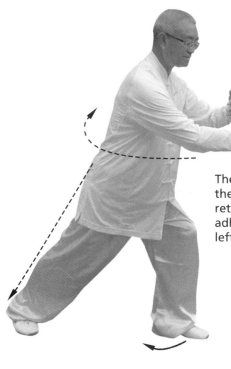

The right heel lifts following the retreating san guan, and retreat with the ball of the foot adhering the ground, to form a left bow stance.

The waist circle turns right led by the elbows, with the torso turning to the right, the left toes turning inward and the right heel turning outward. The right elbow bends horizontally and is sent to the left by following the turning of the torso, with the right palm facing up and the left hand falling to protect the right arm.

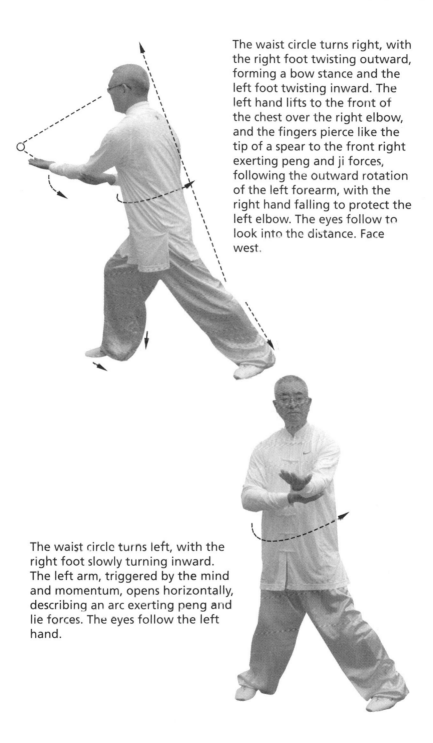

The waist circle turns right, with the right foot twisting outward, forming a bow stance and the left foot twisting inward. The left hand lifts to the front of the chest over the right elbow, and the fingers pierce like the tip of a spear to the front right exerting peng and ji forces, following the outward rotation of the left forearm, with the right hand falling to protect the left elbow. The eyes follow to look into the distance. Face west.

The waist circle turns left, with the right foot slowly turning inward. The left arm, triggered by the mind and momentum, opens horizontally, describing an arc exerting peng and lie forces. The eyes follow the left hand.

The waist circle keeps turning left, with both feet turning, one at a time, on the heels following the torso. The left elbow is bent horizontally and is sent to the right by the turning of the torso, with the palms facing up.

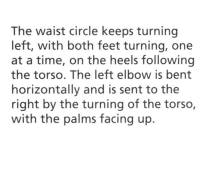

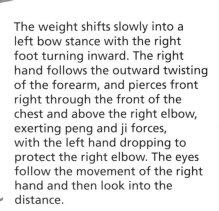

The weight shifts slowly into a left bow stance with the right foot turning inward. The right hand follows the outward twisting of the forearm, and pierces front right through the front of the chest and above the right elbow, exerting peng and ji forces, with the left hand dropping to protect the right elbow. The eyes follow the movement of the right hand and then look into the distance.

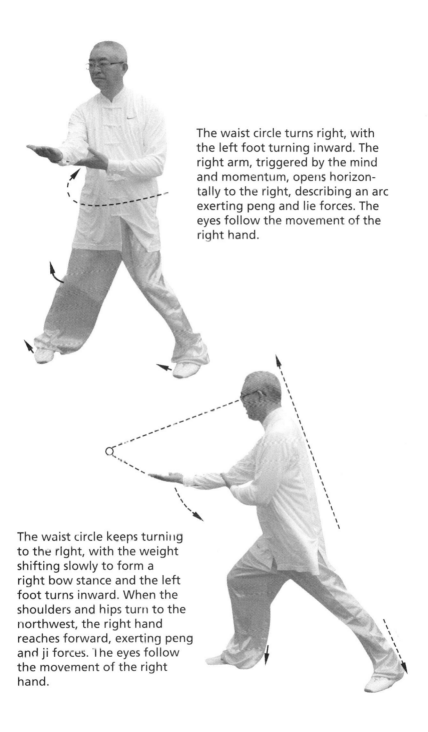

The waist circle turns right, with the left foot turning inward. The right arm, triggered by the mind and momentum, opens horizontally to the right, describing an arc exerting peng and lie forces. The eyes follow the movement of the right hand.

The waist circle keeps turning to the right, with the weight shifting slowly to form a right bow stance and the left foot turns inward. When the shoulders and hips turn to the northwest, the right hand reaches forward, exerting peng and ji forces. The eyes follow the movement of the right hand.

The plumb swings backward, with the arms sinking along a vertical circle, with the palms facing up as if holding an imaginary spear horizontally. Protect the spear in the mind (i.e., hold the imaginary spear as if it were sticking to your palms, followed by drawing back the hands).

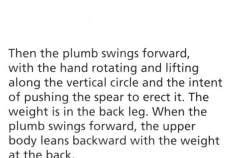

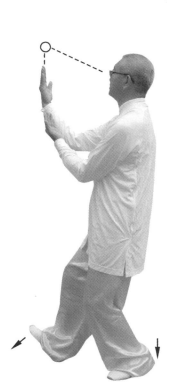

Then the plumb swings forward, with the hand rotating and lifting along the vertical circle and the intent of pushing the spear to erect it. The weight is in the back leg. When the plumb swings forward, the upper body leans backward with the weight at the back.

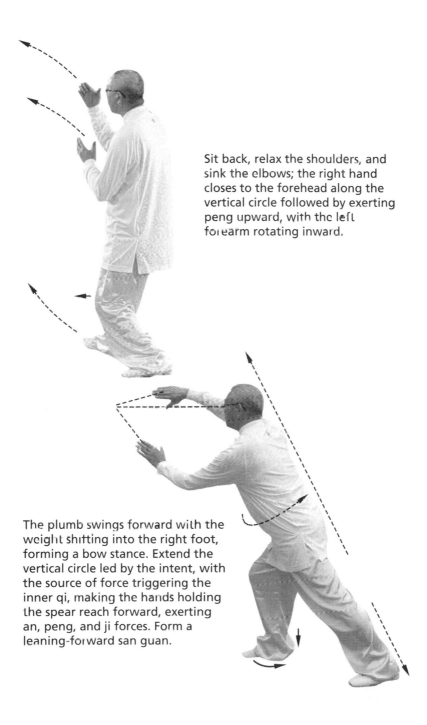

Sit back, relax the shoulders, and sink the elbows; the right hand closes to the forehead along the vertical circle followed by exerting peng upward, with the left forearm rotating inward.

The plumb swings forward with the weight shifting into the right foot, forming a bow stance. Extend the vertical circle led by the intent, with the source of force triggering the inner qi, making the hands holding the spear reach forward, exerting an, peng, and ji forces. Form a leaning-forward san guan.

Right Fair Lady Works the Shuttle

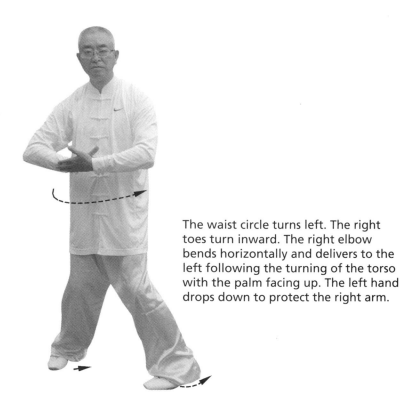

The waist circle turns left. The right toes turn inward. The right elbow bends horizontally and delivers to the left following the turning of the torso with the palm facing up. The left hand drops down to protect the right arm.

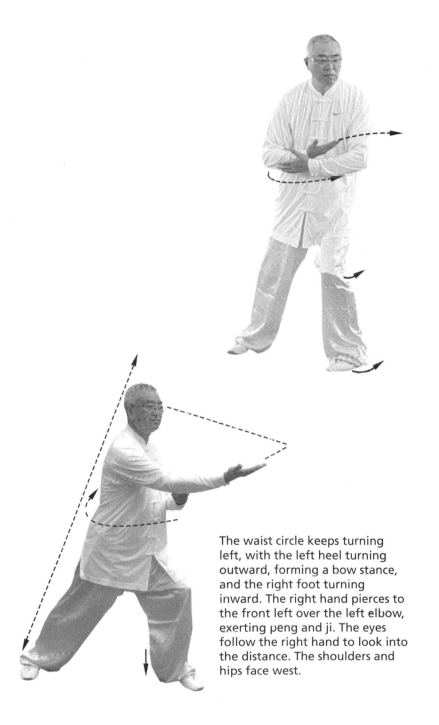

The waist circle keeps turning left, with the left heel turning outward, forming a bow stance, and the right foot turning inward. The right hand pierces to the front left over the left elbow, exerting peng and ji. The eyes follow the right hand to look into the distance. The shoulders and hips face west.

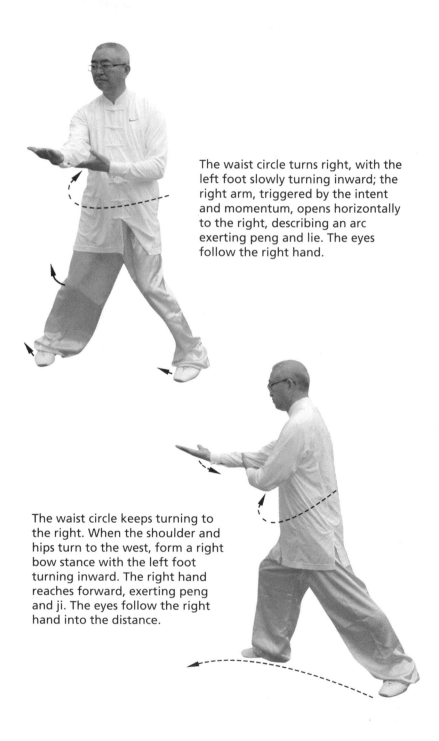

The waist circle turns right, with the left foot slowly turning inward; the right arm, triggered by the intent and momentum, opens horizontally to the right, describing an arc exerting peng and lie. The eyes follow the right hand.

The waist circle keeps turning to the right. When the shoulder and hips turn to the west, form a right bow stance with the left foot turning inward. The right hand reaches forward, exerting peng and ji. The eyes follow the right hand into the distance.

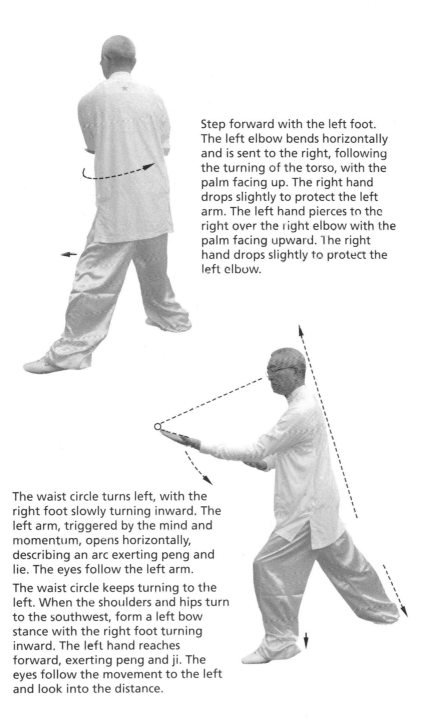

Step forward with the left foot. The left elbow bends horizontally and is sent to the right, following the turning of the torso, with the palm facing up. The right hand drops slightly to protect the left arm. The left hand pierces to the right over the right elbow with the palm facing upward. The right hand drops slightly to protect the left elbow.

The waist circle turns left, with the right foot slowly turning inward. The left arm, triggered by the mind and momentum, opens horizontally, describing an arc exerting peng and lie. The eyes follow the left arm.

The waist circle keeps turning to the left. When the shoulders and hips turn to the southwest, form a left bow stance with the right foot turning inward. The left hand reaches forward, exerting peng and ji. The eyes follow the movement to the left and look into the distance.

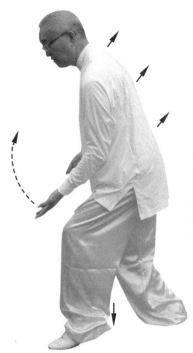

The plumb swings backward, with the arms sinking along a vertical circle, as if holding a spear horizontally with the palms facing up.

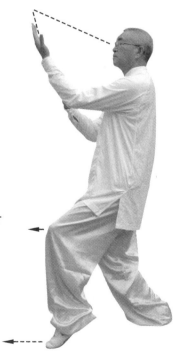

Protect the spear in the mind, followed by drawing back the hands. Then the plumb swings forward, with the hand rotating and lifting along the vertical circle and the intent of pushing the spear to erect it.

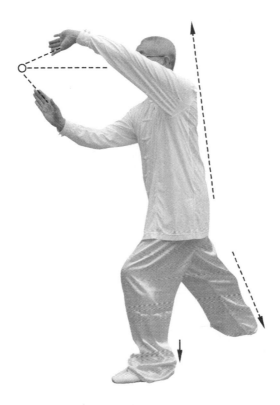

Sit back, relax the shoulders, and sink the elbows. The left hand closes to the forehead along the vertical circle followed by exerting peng upward, with the right forearm rotating inward. The plumb swings forward with the left foot substantializing into a bow stance. Extend the vertical circle led by the intent, with the source of force triggering the inner qi, making the hands holding the spear reach forward, exerting an, peng, and ji. Form a leaning-forward san guan.

15. Downward Posture

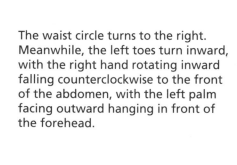

The waist circle turns to the right. Meanwhile, the left toes turn inward, with the right hand rotating inward falling counterclockwise to the front of the abdomen, with the left palm facing outward hanging in front of the forehead.

Form a right bow stance. The right fingers gather to form a hook, with the tip of the hook pointing downward, exerting peng upward to the upper right of the shoulder circle. The left hand supports the right wrist with the index finger, middle finger, and ring finger.

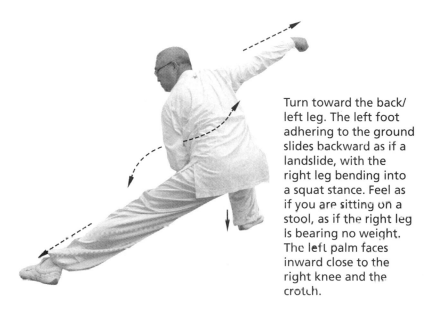

Turn toward the back/
left leg. The left foot
adhering to the ground
slides backward as if a
landslide, with the
right leg bending into
a squat stance. Feel as
if you are sitting on a
stool, as if the right leg
is bearing no weight.
The left palm faces
inward close to the
right knee and the
crotch.

The waist circle turns left, with the
left toes slightly turning outward.
The left fingers point to the front
and the palm is close to the medial
side of the left knee and ankle
piercing forward.

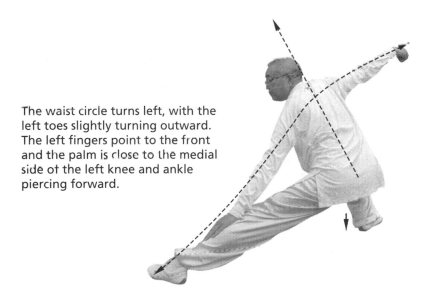

16. Rooster Stands on One Leg

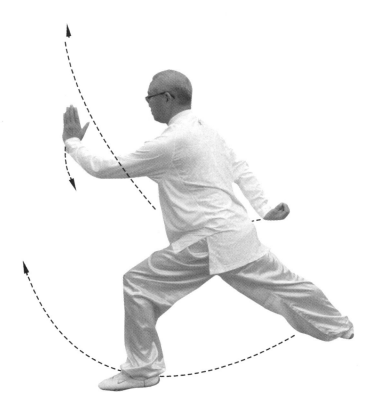

Concentrate the look of the eyes in the direction the left fingers are pointing. The spirit, intent, and qi naturally gather, zigzagging from the cross point of the look and finger direction into the ground continuously, and pierce upper front in an arc, making the left hand and body rise, the right leg lifting naturally, forming a bow stance, the left palm on hold, and the right hook falling to the back of the hips. Face west.

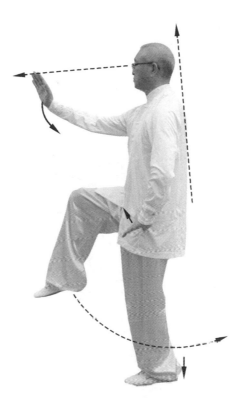

The intent and qi rise, with the inner qi diffusing in the entire body, making the right leg bend and lift. Standing on the left leg, the inner qi diffuses to both arms from the source of force, with the right hook becoming a palm piercing upward, exerting an, peng, and ji. The left hand drops to the left of the hip circle, exerting cai. The energy is full, the inner qi fans out, making the body lean backward.

17. Needle on Sea Floor

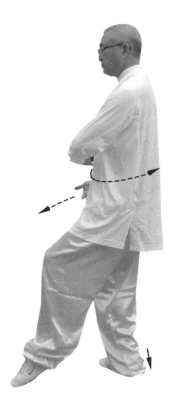

The waist circle turns right, with the right foot stepping to the right back of the left foot. Sit back on the right leg with the left foot touching the ground. The right palm adhering to the small qi ball rotates inward and moves downward. The left one, adhering to the small qi ball, rotates outward and lifts, rotating clockwise until the palms face each other, left on top and right below. Hold the qi mass on the right of the waist circle.

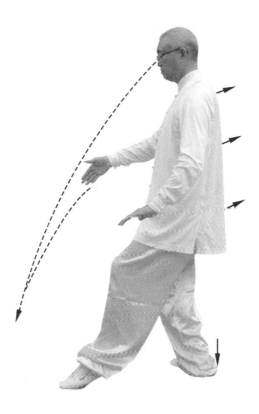

The waist circle turns left. The qi mass rotates counterclockwise, making the left palm rotate outward winding toward the front left of the hip circle, pausing by the left of the hip circle. The right palm rotates inward, facing left, and settles on the right of the waist circle. Lean back with the qi mass diffusing in front of the abdomen as if an "empty valley." (An "empty valley" implies a space so deep that it has the capacity to hold an amount of qi that is beyond imagination.)

The inner qi diffuses to both arms from the source of force. With a compressing and expanding of the mind, the right arm stretches forward, with the qi mass concentrating into a force shooting to the ground in front of the knee.

18. Fan Opens on the Back

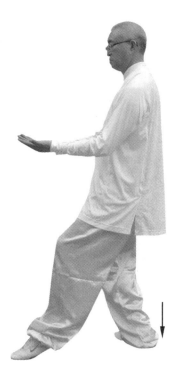

The hands rotate outward and move slightly forward. Imagine receiving the bouncing mass with both hands. The hands are at the same level.

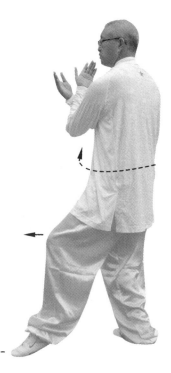

Resume the serenity of the mind, with the body sinking and sitting on the right leg with the left heel on the ground. Bend the elbows with the palms holding back the qi mass. The open hands become fists, crossing in front of the chest, right one on the outside and left one inside, and hold the qi mass in front of the abdomen with the arms.

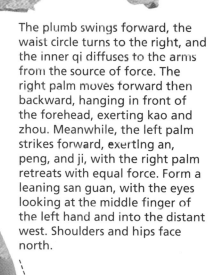

Shift the weight into the left foot, forming a left bow stance. With the fingers of both hands pointing to the upper front, imagine the qi mass embedding into the body. The qi mass goes up to the source of force from the coccyx. The crossing fists separate, becoming open hands and rotating outward, with the elbows on the shoulder circle.

The plumb swings forward, the waist circle turns to the right, and the inner qi diffuses to the arms from the source of force. The right palm moves forward then backward, hanging in front of the forehead, exerting kao and zhou. Meanwhile, the left palm strikes forward, exerting an, peng, and ji, with the right palm retreats with equal force. Form a leaning san guan, with the eyes looking at the middle finger of the left hand and into the distant west. Shoulders and hips face north.

19. Overturn and Throw Fist

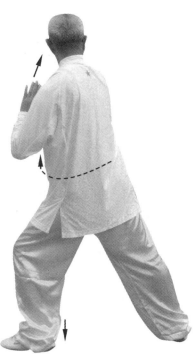

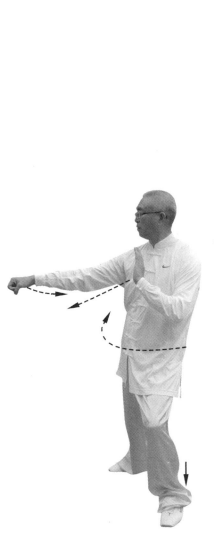

Erect the san guan with the inner qi sinking. The waist circle turns right with the left toes turning inward, forming a pigeon-toed stance. The left hand lifts to the front of the chest with the right palm facing down, grasping the small qi ball and becoming a fist, falling to the waist circle from the forehead, as if grasping the reins on a horse.

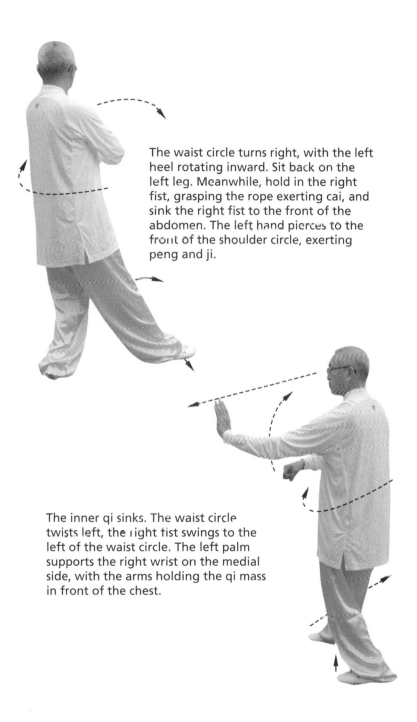

The waist circle turns right, with the left heel rotating inward. Sit back on the left leg. Meanwhile, hold in the right fist, grasping the rope exerting cai, and sink the right fist to the front of the abdomen. The left hand pierces to the front of the shoulder circle, exerting peng and ji.

The inner qi sinks. The waist circle twists left, the right fist swings to the left of the waist circle. The left palm supports the right wrist on the medial side, with the arms holding the qi mass in front of the chest.

The waist circle turns right, the weight shifts left, the right foot moves right, following the turning of the waist. The right fist rotates outward and throws to the right, waist high following the torso, with the eye of the fist facing up. The left hand drops and supports the medial side of the right wrist at the same time. The eyes follow the left hand.

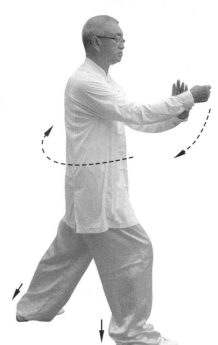

The waist circle twists right, forming a right bow stance. Following the elbow bending and advancing intent, draw in the right fist to the front of the upper abdomen, with the medial side of the fist adhering to the chest and the left palm exerting peng to the front of the shoulder circle.

Whatever move one wants to make, intent comes first. Here one needs to bend the elbow and draw back the right fist with the intent to advance forward, to prepare for the forward movement of the right fist.

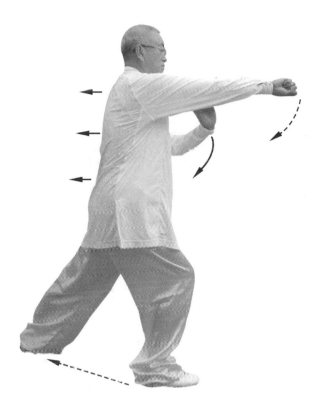

The waist circle turns left with a leaning-back movement, exerting zhou and kao, triggering the right fist moving forward with left rotation and the eye of the fist facing down, exerting peng and ji to the front, following the elbow bending and advancing. The left hand supports the right forearm from the medial side with the index finger, middle finger, and ring finger. Look straight ahead with the shoulders and hips facing east.

20. Retreat, Deflect, Parry, and Punch

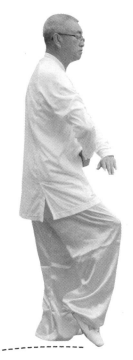

The waist circle quickly turns left. The brisk turning movement causes the body to move with it but only slightly. Substantialize the left foot, with the right fist dropping to protect the crotch, and the left arm settling horizontally on the waist circle.

The waist circle quickly turns right. The plumb swings backward. The right foot retreats. The right fist rotates outward and reaches forward, with the root of the middle finger pointing to the front to "approach the stars," and the left palm gently clinging on the waist circle.

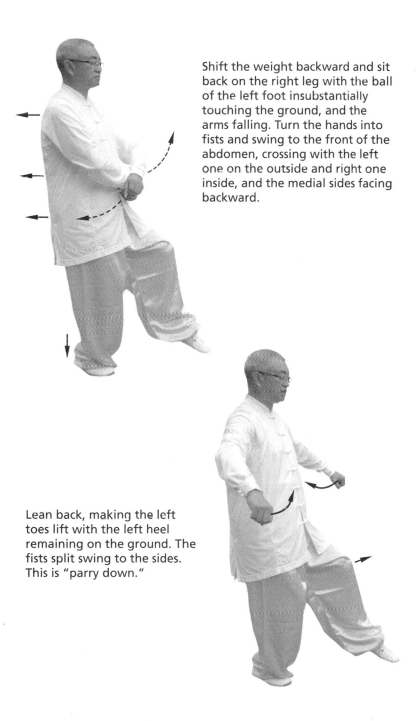

Shift the weight backward and sit back on the right leg with the ball of the left foot insubstantially touching the ground, and the arms falling. Turn the hands into fists and swing to the front of the abdomen, crossing with the left one on the outside and right one inside, and the medial sides facing backward.

Lean back, making the left toes lift with the left heel remaining on the ground. The fists split swing to the sides. This is "parry down."

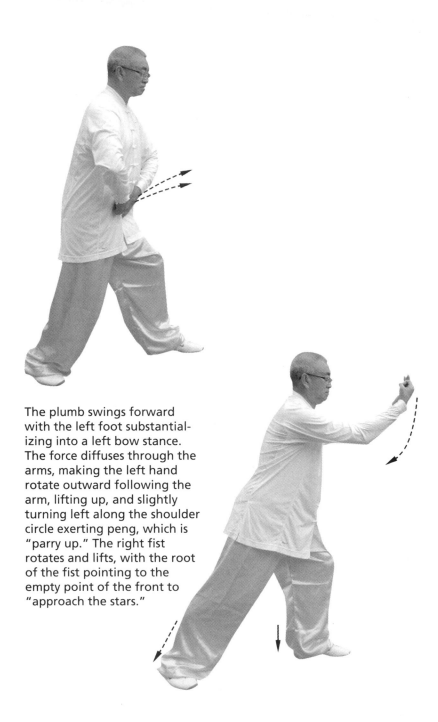

The plumb swings forward with the left foot substantializing into a left bow stance. The force diffuses through the arms, making the left hand rotate outward following the arm, lifting up, and slightly turning left along the shoulder circle exerting peng, which is "parry up." The right fist rotates and lifts, with the root of the fist pointing to the empty point of the front to "approach the stars."

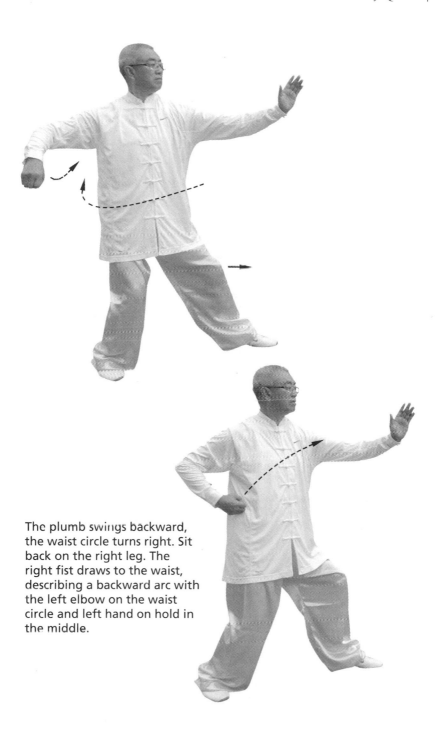

The plumb swings backward, the waist circle turns right. Sit back on the right leg. The right fist draws to the waist, describing a backward arc with the left elbow on the waist circle and left hand on hold in the middle.

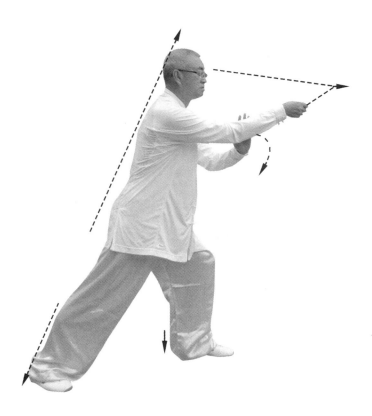

The plumb swings forward, the force reaches to the elbow from the source, triggering the right fist to throw to the front and then dropping, exerting an, peng, and ji, as if beating on water and splashing it around, with the left palm adhering to the medial side of the right arm. Face east.

21. Seal and Close

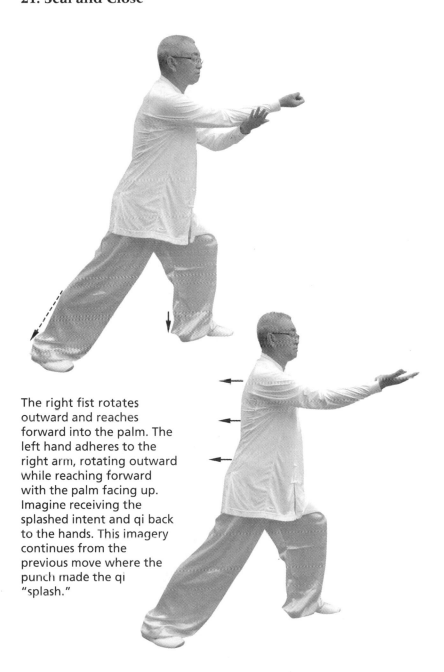

The right fist rotates outward and reaches forward into the palm. The left hand adheres to the right arm, rotating outward while reaching forward with the palm facing up. Imagine receiving the splashed intent and qi back to the hands. This imagery continues from the previous move where the punch made the qi "splash."

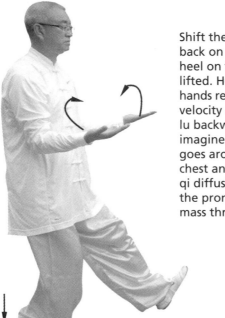

Shift the weight backward and sit back on the right leg, with the left heel on the ground and the toes lifted. Hold the qi mass with both hands reaching forward at constant velocity and equidistance, exerting lu backward, during which imagine a horizontal trident head goes around and penetrates the chest and the back, with the inner qi diffusing into the chest through the prong and introducing a big qi mass through the back.

The intent and qi extend to the front along the sides of the trident, bringing the hands rotating inward and reaching forward, as if the upper body is leaning on the mass.

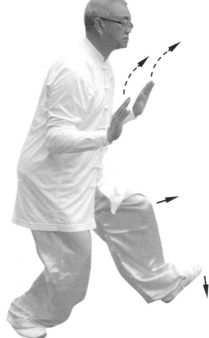

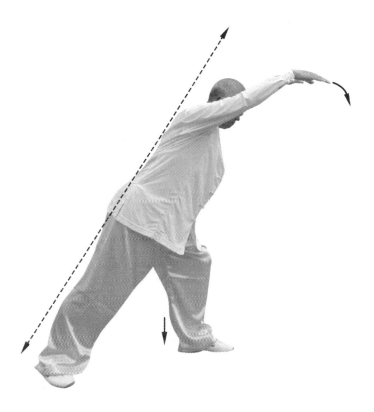

Resume the serenity of the mind, with the left foot substantializing to form a left bow stance. The arms push the big qi mass forward steadily. The qi mass rolls forward. The eyes follow the arms. The shoulders and hips face east.

22. The Cross Hands, Close into Taiji

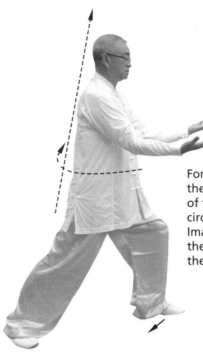

Form a vertical san guan, with the hands falling along the edge of the big qi mass to the waist circle and rotating outward. Imagine holding a big mass with the arms settling horizontally by the sides of the waist circle.

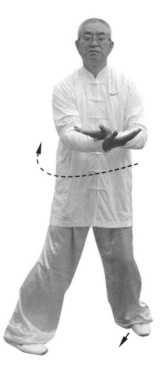

The waist circle turns right, with the left heel turning right 90 degrees. The right foot steps sideways half a step, and the left foot substantializes, forming a squat stance. The left hand slowly pierces to the right, over the right arm, facing up. Hold the qi mass in the arms.

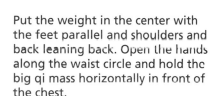

Put the weight in the center with the feet parallel and shoulders and back leaning back. Open the hands along the waist circle and hold the big qi mass horizontally in front of the chest.

The inner qi sinks through the san guan, with the chest held in slightly, forming a horse stance. Imagine swallowing the big qi mass into the chest, with the inner qi diffusing to the hands through the arms from the source of force. Resume the serenity of the mind. Feel an invisible bell caging the body, with the inner qi fanning out from within, making the arms stretch with the back of the hands adhering to the edge of the bell shape.

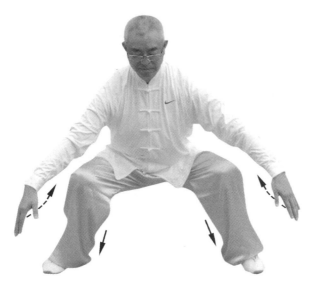

Resume the serenity of the mind. The body drops naturally with the big bell shape lowering, making the legs bend uninten-tionally with the hands adhering to the mouth of the falling bell and crossing in front of the crotch.

The inner qi falls to the ground from the coccyx and bounces onto hands in front of the crotch, making the hands turn inward and lift. Look forward into the distance. When you look forward, the spirit is full. Imagine you are being pulled upward from the top of the head, and it will automatically provide a leading-up power. This is a feeling that develops with practice, and each person will have a different interpretation of the feeling, which itself will change as the practitioner changes.

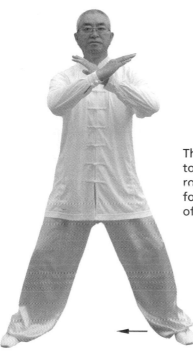

The left foot moves half a step to the right, with the hands rotating inward, following the forearms, drawing to the front of the chest.

Resume the serenity of the mind, with the hands gradually falling, following the sinking of the inner qi, after which the shoulder, waist, and hip circles dissipate.

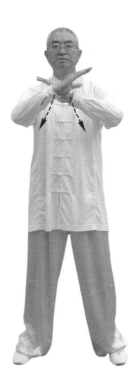

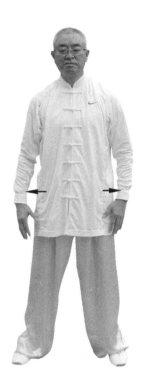

Settle the intent and qi with the inner qi sinking. Imagine the plumb sinking to the middle of the shanks. The hands fall to the front of the hips.

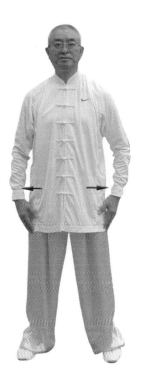

The inner qi rises, making the palms rotate inward, closing in front of the crotch with the palms facing up.

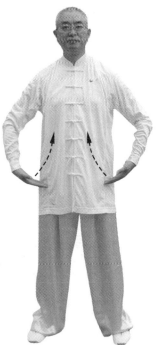

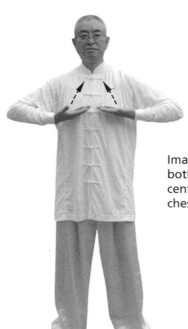

Imagine catching the plumb with both hands and send it to the center of the cross in front of the chest.

The plumb falls from the back of the neck like a falling window shade. The inner qi goes down along the back to the ankles with the spirit exiting, and the hands falling to the sides of the hips.

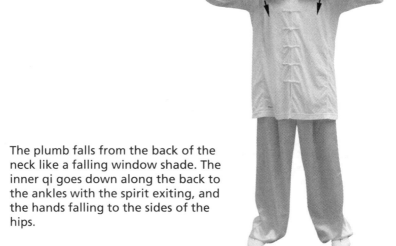

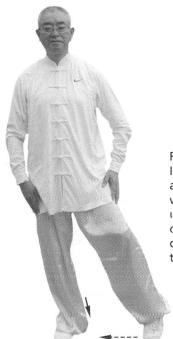

Resume the serenity of the mind. Imagine a dot showing up from a blur at one meter at the front left of the waist, which then separates, moving up and down, with the eyes focusing on the downward movement of the dot, and the left leg moves close to the right one unintentionally.

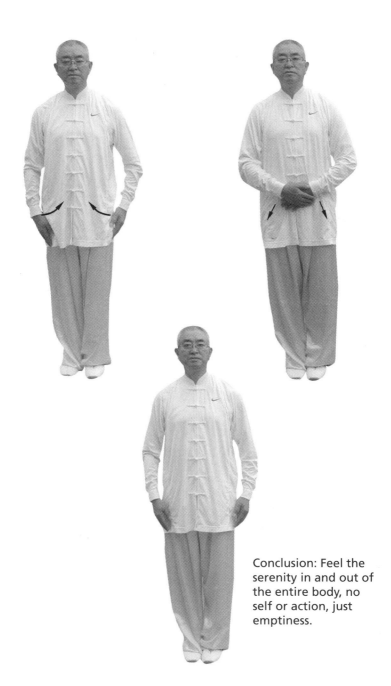

Conclusion: Feel the serenity in and out of the entire body, no self or action, just emptiness.

This book is intended to provide you a simple sequence you can use to practice the mind approach to taijiquan. Even if you prefer a different taiji sequence, the mind approach can be a powerful way to deepen your training. The mind approach will enhance your art and help create more joy in your practice. If you are interested in a richer study of the theories and philosophies behind this approach, please refer to my book *The Mind Inside Tai Chi* (YMAA Publication Center, 2014).

The information I have gathered and offer in this book will assist you whether you are about to enter or have already entered the real world of taijiquan. To get to the essence of taijiquan, remember to study the theories and embrace your practice with an open and peaceful mind.

I thank you for reading my book and I hope I have opened a discussion about our art. It is my sincere wish to share the happiness this approach to taiji practice has brought to me.

> *The way of taiji is the Dao that governs nature.*
> *Carry yin and hold yang when practicing with the mind approach.*
> *Guide qi with the mind, and the body with qi.*
> *Freedom of body and mind.*
> *Unity of human and heaven.*
> *Practice with intent, qi, and form to nurture vigor, qi, and spirit.*
> *Practice relaxation, flexibility, and steadiness to gain peacefulness within the movements.*
> *Develop wisdom and awareness to enjoy a prolonged life.*
> *Instructions of this esoteric approach benefit all people.*

Glossary

an. One of the thirteen basic postures in taijiquan. An means to push or press down. Often it is used as push forward or upward.

baihui (Gv-20). Literally, "hundred meeting." An important acupuncture cavity located on the top of the head. The baihui cavity belongs to the governing vessel du mai. It is also known as "san yang wu hui" (the joint of three yang channels and five vessels), meaning all channels gather here.

bagua. Eight trigrams.

bian. Weak or flat.

cai. Pluck. One of the thirteen basic postures in taijiquan.

cun. A measurement used in acupuncture. It is calculated using the space between the two joints of the thumb or index finger of the individual.

dai mai. Girdle or belt vessel. One of the eight extraordinary vessels. It surrounds the waist and abdominal area in a circle.

dan tian. Elixir field. Locations in the body that store and generate qi. Usually refers to the abdominal area.

dao yin. Literally, "direct and lead." Another name for qigong.

Dao. The "Way." By implication, the "natural way."

dazhui (Gv-14). Acupuncture name for a cavity on the governing vessel. It means "big vertebra."

diu. Lose the touching point.

du mai. Governing vessel. One of the eight extraordinary vessels in Chinese medicine and qigong. The du mai governs the yang channels all over the body. It is the "sea of the yang channels" adjusting the qi and blood of the yang channels.

Duan Baohua. Head of Liang Yi Gongfu. Master to Zhuang Yinghao (Henry Zhuang), the author of this book.

fenshi. Cavity on gallbladder channel.

gongfu. Literally, "energy-time." Any study, learning, or practice that requires a lot of patience, energy, and time to complete. Martial arts are commonly called gongfu.

huantiao. Cavity on gallbladder channel, one on each side of the body, close to the hip joints. "Tiao" means "jump." It commands the lower body movements.

huiyin (Co-1). Literally, "meet yin." An acupuncture cavity belonging to the conception vessel located at the perineum area. It is a critical spot on the ren mai (conception vessel).

ji. Means "to squeeze" or "to press." One of the thirteen basic postures in taijiquan.

jiaji. Cavity at the middle of the shoulder blades.

kang. Resist at the touching point.

kao. Means "bump." One of the thirteen basic postures in taijiquan.

li. Fire.

Li Dao Zi. According to the research of Master Wu Tunan, Li Dao Zi of the Tang dynasty wrote *The Song of Secret Instruction.*

lian. Linking.

liangyi. Yin and yang.

lie. Split or rend. One of the thirteen basic postures in taijiquan.

liu (lu). Rollback. One of the thirteen basic postures in taijiquan.

mingmen. A cavity on the midline of the back waist, in the depression below the spinous process of the second lumbar vertebra. It belongs to the du mai (governing vessel).

nian. Adhering.

peng. Means "ward off." One of the thirteen basic postures in taijiquan.

qi (chi). The general definition of qi is universal energy, including heat, light, and electromagnetic energy. A narrower definition of qi refers to the energy circulating in the human or animal body.

qing. A bell-shaped musical instrument.

qiuxu. Cavity on gallbladder channel.

quan. Fist.

rangu. Cavity on kidney channel.

ren mai. Conception vessel. One of the eight extraordinary vessels in Chinese medicine and qigong. It shares connections with the six yin channels and is called the "sea of the yin channels." It can adjust the qi in the yin channels.

san guan. Three gates. The three gates referred to are weilu, jiaji, and yuzhen.

sanyinjiao. Cavity at the intersection of three channels: spleen, kidney, and liver.

shen ming. Spiritually divine or spiritually enlightened beings.

si xiang. Four forms. Yin and yang give birth to the four forms.

sui. Following.

taiji. Literally, the "grand ultimate." According to Chinese philosophy, taiji is a force that generates two poles, yin and yang, out of wuji (nothingness).

taijiquan (tai chi chuan). Grand ultimate fist. An internal Chinese martial art.

taixi. Cavity on kidney channel.

weilu. Cavity located at the tailbone.

wuji. No extremity. This is the state of undifferentiated emptiness before a beginning.

wushu. Literally, "martial techniques." A common name for the Chinese martial arts.

xuehai. Cavity on spleen channel.

yang. One of the two polarities. The other is yin. In Chinese philosophy, the active, positive, masculine polarity. In Chinese medicine, yang means excessive, too sufficient, overactive, or overheated.

Yang Chengfu (1883–1836 CE). A well-known Yang-style taijiquan master in the 1930s. He was part of the third generation of Yang-style taijiquan practitioners. Yang Luchan was the first generation of the Yang family taijiquan masters, followed by Yang Banhou and Yang Jianhou as the second generation, and Yang Shaohou and Yang Chengfu (the sons of Yang Jianhou) as the third generation.

yang ling quan. Cavity on gallbladder channel.

yin. In Chinese philosophy, the passive, negative, feminine polarity. In Chinese medicine, yin means deficient.

yin ling quan. Cavity on spleen channel, on the medial side of the leg.

ying qi. Nutrient energy.

yongquan (K-1). Cavity on kidney channel, on the bottom of each foot.

yuan qi. Primordial energy.

yuzhen. Jade pillow. Cavity at the base of the skull.

Zen. To endure. The Japanese name for Chan, a school of Buddhism.

zhan. Sticking.

zhongji. Cavity on conception vessel.

zhou. Elbow. To use the elbow to execute techniques in taijiquan. One of the thirteen basic postures.

zong qi. Pectoral energy. Gathering energy.

Index

an force, 26, 30
approaching the stars, 58, 97, 128, 188

baihui, 36
Beijing
  Taijiquan Team of, 7
  Wushu Team of, 4–5
bow stance, 35, 88
  left, 50
  right, 117
Brush Knee and Twist Step
  Left, 66–72, 81–88
  Right, 73–80
Buddhism, 3

cai (tsai) force, 26, 31
Changsha, China, 7
Chinese Academy of Social Sciences
  (CASS), 5, 7
Cloud Hands
  First Open and Close, 126–130
  Second Open and Close, 131–134
  Third Open and Close, 135–139
Commencing Form, 41–46
Cross Hands, Close into Taiji, the,
  194–202
cross in front of chest, the, 22, 141, 144

daimai, 38
dantian, 36, 39, 104
Dao, 3, 6, 36, 203
Downward Posture, 174–175

empty valley, 179

Fair Lady Works the Shuttle, 161–173
  Left, 161–167
  Right, 168–173
Fan Opens on the Back, 180–181
First National Form Sports Contest,
  4–5
foot-shao yin kidney channel, 38
foot-tai yin spleen channel, 38
Forbidden City, 6

gallbladder channel, 38
Grasp the Peacock's Tail
  Left, 104–115
  Right, 116–125

High Pat on Horse, 147–150
Horse stance, 35
huiyin, 38
Hunan Provincial Taijiquan
  Association, 7

intent and qi, 10, 38
  as center, 39
  focus of, 35
  matching flow of, 24–25

jiaji, 17, 18
ji force, 26, 29

kao force, 26, 34
Kick, Left, 159–160

Lao Liu Lu. *See also* Yang-style Lao Liu Lu
  creator of, 2–4
  forms of, 6, 8
  origin of, 1–2
  practicing of, 4
lie force, 26, 32
liu (lu) force, 26, 28
look of the eyes, 24–25

mid-perpendicular, the, 16
mind approach
  key factors of, 9–10
  six points of, 8–9
Mind Inside Tai Chi, The (Zhuang), 9

Needle on Sea Floor, 178–179

Overturn and Throw Fist, 182–185

Parting the Wild Horse's Mane
  Left, 47–53
  Right, 54–59

peng force, 26, 27, 37
People's Sport Publishing House, 5
plumb, the, 16–17
Preparation form, 35–40
Prince Pu Lun Bei Zi, 1, 4
Punch the Ears with Fists, 157–158

qi. *See also* intent and qi
  big qi ball mass, 14–15, 21
  law of, 10
  mass, 14–15
  separation of, 16
  small qi ball, 10, 11–12
  the three circles of, 21
Qing dynasty, 1
Qi Yi, 7

Retreat, Deflect, Parry, and Punch,
    186–190
Retreat and Repulse the Monkey
  Left, 92–98
  Right, 99–103
Rooster Stands on One Leg, 176–177
Rules, 17

san guan
  jaiji of, 17, 18
  leading upward, 18, 19
  leaning forward, 18, 20
  leaning sideways, 18, 19
  retreating, 18, 20
  vertical, 18, 91, 98, 103, 116,
    194
  weilu of, 17, 18, 20
  yuzhen of, 17, 18
Seal and Close, 191–193
serenity of mind, 60, 85, 95, 120, 156,
    157, 196, 201–202
Shanghai, 4
Shou De Martial Arts, 7
Single Whip, 140–146
si zheng shou, 4
source of force, the, 23–24
Splitting Foot, Right, 151–156
Squat stance, 35

Standing Push-Hands, 4
Strum the Lute, 89–91

Taihe Palace, 6
taijiquan, 1, 6
Taijiquan Team, of Beijing, 7
Taijiquan Treatise, 22
Taipei National Martial Arts, 7
three circles of qi, the, 21
True Essence of Yang Style Taijiquan
    (Wei), 2
  initial draft, 5
  organization of, 7
  quotes from, 16, 17
*True Essence of Yang Style Taijiquan
    Internal Power Secret from Yang
    Jianhou* (Wei), 8
*True Essence of Yang Style Taijiquan-
    Lecture Notes* (Wang Yong Quan), 8
*True Essence of Yang Style Taijiquan
    Sequel* (Wei), 7
twenty-four form, 6
twenty-two form, 8, 35

Wang Chong Lu, 1, 2, 4, 5
Wang Yong Quan, 2, 4, 6, 7, 8
weilu, 17, 18, 20
Wei Shu Ren, 2, 7, 16, 17
White Crane Spreads Wings, 60–65
Wudang saber pair, 7
Wuji Stance, 35–36
Wushu Team, of Beijing, 4–5
Wu Style Taijiquan, 26–34

Yang Chengfu, 4
Yang Jian Hou, 1–4, 6
Yang Lu Chan, 4
Yang-style Lao Liu Lu, 1–8
  forms of, 39–40
yin and yang, 8–9, 36, 203
  palms, 25–26, 60
yongquan, 38
yuzhen, 17, 18

Zhou force, 26, 33

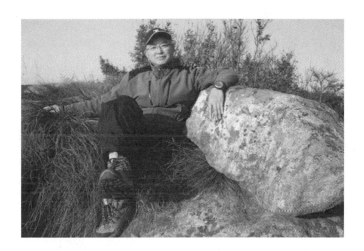

About Henry Zhuang (Zhuang, Yinghao)

Henry Zhuang (Zhuang, Yinghao), born in Shanghai, China, December 11, 1944, is a professional asset and enterprise evaluator and a part-time associate professor at Shanghai Normal University, School of Finance and Business. He loves taijiquan and practices the Buddhadharma. Currently, he is a partner of a professional asset evaluation company, but his lifelong ambition is the promotion of taijiquan culture.

He has studied with Li Zhao Sheng, the creator of meridian circulating taijiquan; Zhu Datong, researcher of taijiquan; Yan Cheng De, a disciple of Zhu Guiting (inheritor of Yang style); Xu Guo Chang (student of Ding De Sheng, disciple of Master Wu Gong Yi), from whom he learned Wu (Gong Yi) style taijiquan. He has acknowledged Shou Guan Shun (student of Zhi Xie Tang, inheritor of Sun-style taijiquan) as his master and been accepted as a disciple by Duan Baohua, the principle master of Liang Yi Dian Xue gongfu.

By the end of the 1990s, concepts of the mind inside the internal power of taijiquan became public. It had been hidden from the public and almost lost. This drove Henry to study the mind approach of internal power with passion. He was fortunate to be instructed by Lang Cheng and Guo Zheng Xun, disciples of Wei Shu Ren (inheritor of The mind approach of internal power of Yang style).

Since 2000, Henry has been giving free lessons on the mind approach of taijiquan to more than sixty business executives, including presidents of prominent companies, partners of the Big Four, bank presidents, and senior managers. For fifteen years, Henry and the taiji fellows have been learning and benefiting from each other. Many of them are now competent teachers of the mind approach. However, teaching face to face has its limitations in spreading the idea of the mind approach. Therefore, from 2012, he started to put his understanding and perceptions into writing books and producing videos.

In May 2013, *The Mind Approach* by Henry Zhuang was published by SDX Joint Publishing Company; during January 2014, the flash of *The Mind Approach of Wu Style Taiji Quan* (Chinese) was published globally in Apple's App Store; in March 2014, the publishing contract of book and ebook on the mind approach was signed between Henry and YMAA Publication Center. IPTV of China Telecom has listed the Mind Approach of Taiji Preservation Coaching as an important content for the Health Channel.

BOOKS FROM YMAA

6 HEALING MOVEMENTS
101 REFLECTIONS ON TAI CHI CHUAN
108 INSIGHTS INTO TAI CHI CHUAN
ADVANCING IN TAE KWON DO
ANALYSIS OF SHAOLIN CHIN NA 2ND ED
ANCIENT CHINESE WEAPONS
ART OF HOJO UNDO
ARTHRITIS RELIEF, 3RD ED.
BACK PAIN RELIEF, 2ND ED.
BAGUAZHANG, 2ND ED.
CARDIO KICKBOXING ELITE
CHIN NA IN GROUND FIGHTING
CHINESE FAST WRESTLING
CHINESE FITNESS
CHINESE TUI NA MASSAGE
CHOJUN
COMPREHENSIVE APPLICATIONS OF SHAOLIN
   CHIN NA
CONFLICT COMMUNICATION
CROCODILE AND THE CRANE: A NOVEL
CUTTING SEASON: A XENON PEARL MARTIAL ARTS
   THRILLER
DEFENSIVE TACTICS
DESHI: A CONNOR BURKE MARTIAL ARTS THRILLER
DIRTY GROUND
DR. WU'S HEAD MASSAGE
DUKKHA HUNGRY GHOSTS
DUKKHA REVERB
DUKKHA, THE SUFFERING: AN EYE FOR AN EYE
DUKKHA UNLOADED
ENZAN: THE FAR MOUNTAIN, A CONNOR BURKE MARTIAL
   ARTS THRILLER
ESSENCE OF SHAOLIN WHITE CRANE
EXPLORING TAI CHI
FACING VIOLENCE
FIGHT BACK
FIGHT LIKE A PHYSICIST
THE FIGHTER'S BODY
FIGHTER'S FACT BOOK
FIGHTER'S FACT BOOK 2
FIGHTING THE PAIN RESISTANT ATTACKER
FIRST DEFENSE
FORCE DECISIONS: A CITIZENS GUIDE
FOX BORROWS THE TIGER'S AWE
INSIDE TAI CHI
KAGE: THE SHADOW, A CONNOR BURKE MARTIAL ARTS
   THRILLER
KATA AND THE TRANSMISSION OF KNOWLEDGE
KRAV MAGA: WEAPON DEFENSES
LITTLE BLACK BOOK OF VIOLENCE
LIUHEBAFA FIVE CHARACTER SECRETS
MARTIAL ARTS ATHLETE
MARTIAL ARTS INSTRUCTION
MARTIAL WAY AND ITS VIRTUES
MASK OF THE KING
MEDITATIONS ON VIOLENCE
MIND/BODY FITNESS
THE MIND INSIDE TAI CHI
MUGAI RYU
NATURAL HEALING WITH QIGONG
NORTHERN SHAOLIN SWORD, 2ND ED.
OKINAWA'S COMPLETE KARATE SYSTEM: ISSHIN RYU
POWER BODY
PRINCIPLES OF TRADITIONAL CHINESE MEDICINE
QIGONG FOR HEALTH & MARTIAL ARTS 2ND ED.

QIGONG FOR LIVING
QIGONG FOR TREATING COMMON AILMENTS
QIGONG MASSAGE
QIGONG MEDITATION: EMBRYONIC BREATHING
QIGONG MEDITATION: SMALL CIRCULATION
QIGONG, THE SECRET OF YOUTH: DA MO'S CLASSICS
QUIET TEACHER: A XENON PEARL MARTIAL ARTS
   THRILLER
RAVEN'S WARRIOR
ROOT OF CHINESE QIGONG, 2ND ED.
SCALING FORCE
SENSEI: A CONNOR BURKE MARTIAL ARTS THRILLER
SHIHAN TE: THE BUNKAI OF KATA
SHIN GI TAI: KARATE TRAINING FOR BODY, MIND, AND
   SPIRIT
SIMPLE CHINESE MEDICINE
SIMPLE QIGONG EXERCISES FOR HEALTH, 3RD ED.
SIMPLIFIED TAI CHI CHUAN, 2ND ED
SIMPLIFIED TAI CHI FOR BEGINNERS
SOLO TRAINING
SOLO TRAINING 2
SUDDEN DAWN: THE EPIC JOURNEY OF BODHIDHARMA
SUNRISE TAI CHI
SUNSET TAI CHI
SURVIVING ARMED ASSAULTS
TAE KWON DO: THE KOREAN MARTIAL ART
TAEKWONDO BLACK BELT POOMSAE
TAEKWONDO: A PATH TO EXCELLENCE
TAEKWONDO: ANCIENT WISDOM FOR THE MODERN
   WARRIOR
TAEKWONDO: DEFENSES AGAINST WEAPONS
TAEKWONDO: SPIRIT AND PRACTICE
TAO OF BIOENERGETICS
TAI CHI BALL QIGONG: FOR HEALTH AND MARTIAL ARTS
TAI CHI BALL WORKOUT FOR BEGINNERS
TAI CHI BOOK
TAI CHI CHIN NA: THE SEIZING ART OF TAI CHI CHUAN,
   2ND ED.
TAI CHI CHUAN CLASSICAL YANG STYLE, 2ND ED.
TAI CHI CHUAN MARTIAL APPLICATIONS
TAI CHI CHUAN MARTIAL POWER, 3RD ED.
TAI CHI CONNECTIONS
TAI CHI DYNAMICS
TAI CHI QIGONG, 3RD ED.
TAI CHI SECRETS OF THE ANCIENT MASTERS
TAI CHI SECRETS OF THE WU & LI STYLES
TAI CHI SECRETS OF THE WU STYLE
TAI CHI SECRETS OF THE YANG STYLE
TAI CHI SWORD: CLASSICAL YANG STYLE, 2ND ED.
TAI CHI SWORD FOR BEGINNERS
TAI CHI WALKING
TAIJIQUAN THEORY OF DR. YANG, JWING-MING
TENGU: THE MOUNTAIN GOBLIN, A CONNOR BURKE MAR-
   TIAL ARTS THRILLER
TIMING IN THE FIGHTING ARTS
TRADITIONAL CHINESE HEALTH SECRETS
TRADITIONAL TAEKWONDO
WAY OF KATA
WAY OF KENDO AND KENJITSU
WAY OF SANCHIN KATA
WAY TO BLACK BELT
WESTERN HERBS FOR MARTIAL ARTISTS
WILD GOOSE QIGONG
WOMAN'S QIGONG GUIDE
XINGYIQUAN

continued on next page . . .

DVDS FROM YMAA

ADVANCED PRACTICAL CHIN NA IN-DEPTH

ANALYSIS OF SHAOLIN CHIN NA

BAGUAZHANG: EMEI BAGUAZHANG

CHEN STYLE TAIJIQUAN

CHIN NA IN-DEPTH COURSES 1—4

CHIN NA IN-DEPTH COURSES 5—8

CHIN NA IN-DEPTH COURSES 9—12

FACING VIOLENCE: 7 THINGS A MARTIAL ARTIST MUST
    KNOW

FIVE ANIMAL SPORTS

JOINT LOCKS

KNIFE DEFENSE: TRADITIONAL TECHNIQUES AGAINST A
    DAGGER

KUNG FU BODY CONDITIONING 1

KUNG FU BODY CONDITIONING 2

KUNG FU FOR KIDS

KUNG FU FOR TEENS

INFIGHTING

LOGIC OF VIOLENCE

MERIDIAN QIGONG

NEIGONG FOR MARTIAL ARTS

NORTHERN SHAOLIN SWORD : SAN CAI JIAN, KUN WU
    JIAN, QI MEN JIAN

QIGONG MASSAGE

QIGONG FOR HEALING

QIGONG FOR LONGEVITY

QIGONG FOR WOMEN

SABER FUNDAMENTAL TRAINING

SAI TRAINING AND SEQUENCES

SANCHIN KATA: TRADITIONAL TRAINING FOR KARATE
    POWER

SHAOLIN KUNG FU FUNDAMENTAL TRAINING: COURSES
    1 & 2

SHAOLIN LONG FIST KUNG FU: BASIC SEQUENCES

SHAOLIN LONG FIST KUNG FU: INTERMEDIATE SE-
    QUENCES

SHAOLIN LONG FIST KUNG FU: ADVANCED SEQUENCES 1

SHAOLIN LONG FIST KUNG FU: ADVANCED SEQUENCES 2

SHAOLIN SABER: BASIC SEQUENCES

SHAOLIN STAFF: BASIC SEQUENCES

SHAOLIN WHITE CRANE GONG FU BASIC TRAINING:
    COURSES 1 & 2

SHAOLIN WHITE CRANE GONG FU BASIC TRAINING:
    COURSES 3 & 4

SHUAI JIAO: KUNG FU WRESTLING

SIMPLE QIGONG EXERCISES FOR ARTHRITIS RELIEF

SIMPLE QIGONG EXERCISES FOR BACK PAIN RELIEF

SIMPLIFIED TAI CHI CHUAN: 24 & 48 POSTURES

SIMPLIFIED TAI CHI FOR BEGINNERS 48

SUNRISE TAI CHI

SUNSET TAI CHI

SWORD: FUNDAMENTAL TRAINING

TAEKWONDO KORYO POOMSAE

TAI CHI BALL QIGONG: COURSES 1 & 2

TAI CHI BALL QIGONG: COURSES 3 & 4

TAI CHI BALL WORKOUT FOR BEGINNERS

TAI CHI CHUAN CLASSICAL YANG STYLE

TAI CHI CONNECTIONS

TAI CHI ENERGY PATTERNS

TAI CHI FIGHTING SET

TAI CHI PUSHING HANDS: COURSES 1 & 2

TAI CHI PUSHING HANDS: COURSES 3 & 4

TAI CHI SWORD: CLASSICAL YANG STYLE

TAI CHI SWORD FOR BEGINNERS

TAI CHI SYMBOL: YIN YANG STICKING HANDS

TAIJI & SHAOLIN STAFF: FUNDAMENTAL TRAINING

TAIJI CHIN NA IN-DEPTH

TAIJI 37 POSTURES MARTIAL APPLICATIONS

TAIJI SABER CLASSICAL YANG STYLE

TAIJI WRESTLING

UNDERSTANDING QIGONG 1: WHAT IS QI? • HUMAN QI
    CIRCULATORY SYSTEM

UNDERSTANDING QIGONG 2: KEY POINTS • QIGONG
    BREATHING

UNDERSTANDING QIGONG 3: EMBRYONIC BREATHING

UNDERSTANDING QIGONG 4: FOUR SEASONS QIGONG

UNDERSTANDING QIGONG 5: SMALL CIRCULATION

UNDERSTANDING QIGONG 6: MARTIAL QIGONG
    BREATHING

WHITE CRANE HARD & SOFT QIGONG

WUDANG KUNG FU: FUNDAMENTAL TRAINING

WUDANG SWORD

WUDANG TAIJIQUAN

XINGYIQUAN

YANG TAI CHI FOR BEGINNERS

YMAA 25 YEAR ANNIVERSARY DVD

more products available from . . .

YMAA Publication Center, Inc. 楊氏東方文化出版中心

1-800-669-8892 • info@ymaa.com • www.ymaa.com